WISE

Elaine Harris is a social scientist, yoga therapist, reiki practitioner, blogger and mother. She is living and experiencing the rite of passage to midlife at the time of writing this book. Elaine has two children and lives in Wicklow with her husband, Damien Duff.

WISE

FINDING MEANING, PURPOSE & INNER POWER IN MIDLIFE

Elaine Harris

Gill Books

Gill Books
Hume Avenue
Park West
Dublin 12
www.gillbooks.ie

Gill Books is an imprint of M.H. Gill and Co.

978 07171 9722 4

Designed by iota (iota-books.ie)
Illustrations by Tara O'Brien
Edited by Gráinne Treanor
Proofread by Ciara McNee
Printed and bound by BZ Graf, Poland
This book is typeset in Galliard with Le Havre display.

*The paper used in this book comes from the
wood pulp of sustainably managed forests.*

A CIP catalogue record for this book is
available from the British Library.

This book is not intended as a substitute
for the medical advice of a physician.
The reader should consult a doctor or mental
health professional if they feel it necessary.

Some names and identifying details have been
changed to protect the privacy of the people
involved.

5 4 3 2 1

For Darcy and Woody,
my greatest teachers.

Contents

Introduction

Five years ago, at 41 years of age, I found myself burnt out. The embarrassing thing was that I was teaching hundreds of children and adults each week how to relax and find inner peace in my role as a yoga teacher and therapist – yet, ironically, I was stressed out and exhausted to the point of wanting to escape my own life. And that is exactly what I did.

In 2018, my husband, Damien, was offered a job in the UK. He had recently retired from playing professional soccer and was transitioning into coaching players. Knowing that retiring could be a notoriously difficult time for ex-players, I felt that this new job would be great opportunity for him. Selfishly, I also saw it as my chance to escape my – completely self-inflicted – over-burdened routine. Having lived a pretty nomadic life, moving homes almost 20 times, I was more comfortable uprooting the whole family rather than confronting my own inner issues. So, on the first day of the new year, we took the ferry to Scotland.

In Glasgow, with our children in a new school and Damien extremely busy in his new role, I slowed everything right down, teaching just two yoga classes a week. Without the distraction of being busy, I found that I was forced into a period of reflection and introspection. This involved a deepening of my practice of yoga and meditation, expanding my study of yoga therapy and exploring healing modalities such as reiki, sacred dance and emotional freedom technique (EFT), as well as reading numerous books and spiritual texts and listening to personal growth podcasts. It was also a time of immense creative expression and I found myself inspired to write and make art.

My self-imposed retreat elongated as the world went into lockdown. This time of slow living coincided with my crossing the threshold into midlife – a critical rite of passage in a woman's life. Every woman who reaches that stage will experience the turning point to midlife, but for each of us it might look very different. For me, I felt the need to make sense of what I had already experienced and mine the wisdom gained from my life so far. It became clearer to me that I had been living in ways that were out of alignment with who I was, or who I was in the process of becoming – and what I came here to do. Compounded by a sense of urgency to become more authentic, my awareness expanded to see the parts of myself that needed re-parenting. Gaining my integrity manifested in a shift in the dynamics of some of my relationships and friendships. At times this process felt untethering, vulnerable, exposing and often very lonely – but it was absolutely worth every challenging step to recover myself and step into my authenticity.

I believe that each of us has been tasked with an individual quest or a purpose, and we are born with unique gifts and talents that support us on our mission. Every life experience that we have, even our most painful ones, is a chance for learning and gaining insight that we can embody as wisdom to help us on our quest. Our means of self-expression, and to whom we impart these nuggets of wisdom, will also be unique to each of us. The inner work that we do as we move into midlife, and our commitment to this work, facilitates us stepping into our birth right to become wise women.

This is what nudged me to create this book – a guide to help you make sense of your own journey into midlife. This passage requires that we contemplate those things that might be stopping us from carrying our wisdom forward and sharing it with those coming behind us for the greater good. This is how we become the fullest expression of ourselves.

How smooth or rocky this transition will be for each of us is influenced by how we live our lives now. In our modern Western world, many of us have adopted a way of living that is out of sync with who we really are, and have accepted this way of life as normal without questioning it. We can witness the consequences of this in the physical, energetic, mental, emotional and spiritual suffering experienced by so many women all over the

Western world, and yet we continue pushing ourselves to keep up with the expectations and demands of modern life, sacrificing our wholeness – the unity of the body, mind and spirit.

Our modern lifestyles are structured, rigid and linear, even though our indigenous female nature is rhythmic and cyclical. We are fluid, our energy is undulating, our emotions and feelings are transient, and we are influenced by the flow of the seasons in nature. We have our monthly dance with the cycles of hormonal fluctuations. And from birth through to death we are initiated into many different stages of our lifespan – puberty, pregnancy and motherhood (for some of us), transitioning into midlife and becoming an elder and then an ancestor. Living in a way that does not consider all these seasons and rhythms – in fact, often ignoring them entirely – we move way out of balance with who we are. Our wholeness relies on an intricate balance or homeostasis, and when this unity is compromised, we become fragmented and disconnected from our authenticity, intention and purpose on this planet.

But could we stop to consider the possibility that there might be a different way to live – even a better way to live that is in alignment with our natural human cycles, the cycle of life and the rhythm of the earth? Midlife is a particularly complex life stage for modern women. As we begin to transition, we experience hormonal changes that diminish our fertility, and we are provided with profound opportunities to use our life-giving energy to birth something new. This can be the rebirthing of ourselves into becoming who we are truly meant to be in this lifetime. Moving into midlife, we are no longer objectified for our youthful looks, and although this may be a loss we need to grieve, it can actually help us to remember that we are more than our physical bodies. Nature guides us to direct our awareness inwards to discover our inner power – a pool of infinite wisdom. This is the journey through our inner landscape to meet our wise woman – a rite of passage that is underappreciated.

But many of the values of our modern world compound the uncertainty and challenges we women experience at this liminal time in our lives. We are culturally conditioned to continue as normal while undergoing deeply personal shifts, hormonal symptoms and even spiritual transformation. Without a safe container of space and time to assimilate and integrate the changes happening at all levels of our being, we are expected to carry on regardless. Overwhelmed by this struggle between the outer world and our inner landscape, we may start to feel like there is something wrong with us, punishing ourselves by believing that we are to blame for not keeping up with the pace of life or for not being able to adapt well enough to all that we must attend to.

And all the while the call to rebirth ourselves grows stronger. This feels like an inner uprising asking us to pay attention. Our dreams become wildly vivid. We may recall old memories and wounds buried deep within, telling us that now is the time to help them heal so they can no longer hurt us. We may feel a yearning for more soulful experiences in our life and a desire for more meaningful connections, and we may feel called to express ourselves in untried ways. During this process of awakening, we may slowly begin to recognise that we are living in a way that does not support or honour all that we are. We are then left with a choice: to stay on the same path, pushing and pulling, contorting who we are to conform to the norms of our modern culture; or to stop and come home to ourselves, embrace our wholeness, and create a new way of living.

Our rite of passage into midlife requires deep self-nurturing, kindness and healing so that we can be the most whole version of ourselves. It requires radical self-love and acceptance. If we continue wasting our energy on self-loathing, doubting that we are enough, we block ourselves in making this transition from wisdom seeker to wisdom keeper. When we start to trust ourselves, connect with our intuition, and shift our consciousness, we awaken to our wisdom.

My hope is that this book will help you on this journey of awakening, and that it will support you to take a deep dive to become all that you are. You may not share all aspects of my worldview or philosophies, but I invite you to be open to elements that might resonate with your own experience and to consider the possibility that these may be of some value to you on your own journey. As you read through the chapters, you can join me in an exploration of all the layers of our being. Each chapter contains one or more practices to help you do this, as well as a case study showing how an individual has experienced this journey in their own lives. 'Pearls of wisdom' at the end of each chapter provide a concise summary to remind you of the key themes of the chapter and to act as a quick refresher to dip into from time to time.

By working through the body, the breath, the energy centres, the mind and the heart, and by exploring the meaningful connections in our lives, we can tap into the wisdom of midlife and attune to the whispers of life. Then we can come to know our gifts and purpose for being here. Finding the courage to take action, we can step into our power and honour the wise presence we can be in the world. When we answer nature's call to rise up as wise women, we offer so much to the world. But we first need to come home to ourselves. By pausing and slowing down to respect our intrinsic rhythms, and by simplifying our lives to allow more joy and pleasure, we unearth our sacred wisdom. As each one of us awakens to this inner work, we shift the landscape of the outer world.

This is important work, and we must take care of ourselves so that we can make this journey safely. You may wish to create a *women's circle* as you work through the book. This might be a community of women coming together to support each other through dialogue and connection. You may already have a group of women that you meet up with, perhaps for a book club, and it might organically feel like a good fit to do this work together. Women of all ages can be a support. Our elders will have already navigated this journey and can offer the wisdom of their lived experience. Younger women will have fresh perspectives and creative ideas that can ignite and inspire us to honour our potential.

Our journey will be their journey eventually, and in this sharing circle with our younger sisters, they have the opportunity to prepare and learn from the challenges we face during our transition.

Whichever way you choose to approach the book – either on your own or as part of a group – please be kind to yourself. Create a safe and comfortable cocoon as you work through the chapters. Mother yourself as you would a child, offering a sense of safety and protection. Allow yourself to accept all the parts of yourself that you discover along the way. Know that all parts are welcome and that you are enough. Find time for relaxation and self-care rituals, and above all else practise compassion for all that you have been and all that you are becoming.

From my heart to yours,
Elaine

CHAPTER ONE

Wise Women

"*You are either losing your mind or gaining your soul.*"

JULIA CAMERON

My mother is 70 years of age. Thankfully, she is very healthy and independent. She is adventurous and full of life. With plenty of friends, she has a diary so full of social plans that my sisters and I joke that we need an appointment to see her. In saying that, if any of us asks her for a favour, she will drop everything to be there, or at the very least she will volunteer my father to help. Like many women, she is selfless and puts the needs of others first, often at a cost to her own well-being. Research shows that we become more altruistic as we age. In fact, on average, older people are kinder and genuinely more interested in the welfare of others than are their younger peers.[1] This makes sense, as we are often less consumed by the duties that kept us busy when we were younger – work, childcare, managing a busy household – and we may therefore have more time for others. As we grow and evolve, we also lose some of the self-consciousness that keeps us more narrowly focused on ourselves. And as we gain lived experience, we may have fulfilled some of our own needs, allowing us to focus on the noble act of helping others. When our tank is full, we can give to others.

Our needs matter

Over 70 years ago, Abraham Maslow, an American psychologist, introduced the world to his theory of human motivation. He proposed that when we have satisfied our basic human needs, we can become kinder and more benevolent towards each other. He described a 'hierarchy of needs' model that identifies core human needs across six categories: our physiological needs; our need for safety and security; our need for love and belonging; our need for esteem; and our need for self-actualisation and transcendence. Maslow said the first four groups of core needs are deficiency needs, meaning that when these aren't met our well-being is encumbered. He viewed the top two categories – self-actualisation and transcendence – as needs that support our personal growth. Maslow's theory proposed that our deficiency needs must be addressed before we can move up the hierarchal ladder and cultivate our personal growth.[2]

Maslow's hierarchy of needs

TRANSCENDENCE
Supports our highest human potential, that is, elevates
our consciousness, transcends our ego. We lose our self-
consciousness, experiencing flow states and spiritual
connection that are part of a higher power. We have a feeling
of oneness with each other, nature, all species and the universe.

SELF-ACTUALISATION
Supports us reaching our potential as a person,
that is, education, training, developing our
gifts and talents, helping others.

ESTEEM
Supports our self-esteem, self-respect,
self-confidence and independence.

LOVE AND BELONGING
Supports our social needs, that is, supportive relationships
with family, friends, partners, colleagues. We have a sense
of belonging to community and social groups.

SAFETY AND SECURITY
Supports us to feel safe and secure, protected from
violence and theft, and to have financial stability.

PHYSIOLOGICAL NEEDS
Supports our physical well-being, like food, water,
shelter, warmth, clothing, rest, access to healthcare.

As we know, life is not static. It is dynamic, and the circumstances of our lives change and fluctuate, impacting our deficiency and growth needs. Some of us may have accumulated a lot of material wealth – we may have the big house, a nice car, lots of expensive clothes – but have spent less of our lives expanding our personal growth and spiritual dimension. We may know many people whose primary needs are under threat but who are deeply spiritual, altruistic and connected to nature.

In this regard, our needs may be less linear or hierarchical than the model suggests, and, in reality, more circular. Nevertheless, Maslow's model is useful in showing us the multifaceted nature of our being, and it is useful for our own self-exploration. As we transition to midlife, we are called to get to know ourselves better and reflect on how we live our lives. Socrates, considered to be one of the wisest men in Ancient Greece, is believed to have said that the unexamined life is a life not worth living. The passage to midlife presents the opportunity to examine our lives, to look at where we have been, and to explore where we are going. When we look at the hierarchy of needs and apply it to ourselves, we can see which of our core human needs we feel have been met and which outstanding needs we feel are yet to be realised. It can show us which core set of needs are most important to us and which set(s) we pay less attention to. This can help us to understand not only ourselves but also our human potential.

PRACTICE: Applying the hierarchy of needs to your own life

Look at the diagram showing Maslow's hierarchy of needs on page 5. Consider the following core group of needs: physiological, safety and security, love and belonging, esteem, self-actualisation and transcendence. Reflect on your own life:

○ What needs do you feel are addressed in your life?
○ What needs do you feel are not yet fulfilled in your life?
○ What is the main reason they are not yet fulfilled?
○ In your life now, which needs feel the most important to you?
○ In your life now, which needs feel the least important to you?

As our deficiency needs are met, we are able to focus on what is important for us and for humanity. By midlife, a great many of us in the Western world feel more secure with our physical and safety needs met, and we can therefore have a wider perspective and a greater desire to connect with one another and to develop the qualities of kindness and empathy. This natural stage of life is guiding us to focus on our personal growth needs – to self-actualise and find transcendence.

The responsibility of privilege

Many of us, by virtue of our geography and circumstances, may already be privileged with a higher standard of living relative to others. With our privilege, we have a responsibility to our sisters and brothers who do not have equal access to their fundamental human rights and whose basic needs are not yet met. We must do what we can from our place of privilege to have a more positive impact on this world. There is no time to wait for the change we want to see in the world – *we* must be the change-makers. The Dalai Lama is said to have prophesied that the world will be saved by Western women.[3] This is not because we are better than anyone else, but because of the combination of privilege and the unique qualities that women can bring to the world when we connect with our inner power.

In a context in which our natural world is under threat, we need to change to become worthy guardians of the earth and of each other. It will take compassionate leadership to shift and transform in order to heal the fractures in our world. The wisdom of women is an underutilised resource in our current world. We don't have time to wait for the system to change and invite us to the table. As women, we must all do our part, taking responsibility for the contribution that we can make and creating spaces to express our wisdom and disseminate it to the world. If we see gaps where the wisdom of women is missing, we must become the trailblazers, paving the way for the next generation of women. This might mean answering a call to become a leader in your community – getting involved in advocacy, policy-making or entering local politics. It could mean using your creative talents to express your wisdom through entrepreneurship, technology or a piece of music, writing, art or film.

Great transformation starts with small right actions

No one is too small, too young or too old to make a difference. Each of us has a particular purpose and role here on the planet at this specific time in history. Just as the tiniest creature in the natural world has an intricate role in the ecosystem, so each of us has been placed here with a mission that will have a ripple effect in the wider world. Our function now, in midlife, is to allow our potential as wise women to unfold. We are ready with the necessary knowledge and wisdom of lived experience to fulfil the unique role that we came here to do, and it is time to courageously share our gifts so that we can be impactful. As we approach midlife, some of us experience a strengthening of the call of our soul to create the impact we came to make. It may manifest as a deep yearning that becomes impossible to ignore. It may speak to us as physical sensations or waves of deep feelings and emotions until we begin to pay attention. Once we begin to answer the call to uncover who we really are, we embark on a rapid journey of personal growth and transformation.

The journey home

At this time in our lives, we are called on a quest – a journey through the depths of our layers to undo much of what we have been conditioned to believe about ourselves and the world – so that we may find the unique treasure buried deep inside and awaken our inner power. The preface of transformation can feel like a period of intense upheaval and uncertainty, which can be disturbing, especially if we are not prepared, As we do the work, however, we come to learn that our power has been with us all along. Much like Dorothy in *The Wizard of Oz* or Santiago the shepherd in Paulo Coelho's *The Alchemist*, we have everything that we need inside of us.[4]

This can come as a surprise if we have spent a great deal of our lives focused externally, looking to find meaning, power and purpose outside of ourselves. When we look outside of ourselves, we become fragmented, as the external world is so divided. It takes journeying inwards through our inner landscape to return to our sense of wholeness. The work to go inwards is not easy and can feel very unsettling. After spending so much time looking out, we might be afraid to finally meet ourselves. We may not be sure that we will actually like what we see. But if we avoid this journey, we will never come to know who we truly are and why we are here – or achieve our truest potential. Please rest assured that it is possible and probable that you might very much like who you meet along the way – your true self – as you journey through this rite of passage and see the difference you can bring to the world.

How did we get lost?

One day during school holidays, while I was walking through the woods with my kids, who were 10 and 11, a little boy of about three years of age came running up to us and started telling us all about himself and what magic tools he had in his backpack. His father came up behind him and began to apologise for his son, Alex, saying that the little boy had been out of preschool for so long he was missing talking to different people.

The older kids loved the three-year-old's imagination and got a great kick out of recalling his chats for the rest of the day. It got us thinking about that beautiful openness of young children, where they feel confident to speak to strangers – as W.B. Yeats called them, the friends they have not yet met.[5] It is when we start to worry about what others might think of us that we begin to become more closed. If the message we receive from our family, school, community and the wider world is that it is not safe to be ourselves, then we start to wear masks to project an image of ourselves that we believe the outside world will accept. Compounding this, we are also socialised into roles that are normalised for our biological sex according to our families, wider society and culture. This process of masking is born out of a perceived need to self-protect. We become champion chameleons, able to adapt and change to try to fit in with the accepted values of our world. As we try to mirror how we think the world wants us to be, we become untethered from who we really are.

Yin and yang – the balance of life

The natural world relies on a delicate balance between a sum of interconnected parts that make up the whole. We are each individually part of the natural world, so we influence this balance. Internally, we are each made up of a system of inner parts that are interdependent, and which also need balance to function harmoniously. Within both the macro (the world) and the micro (us individually), life is sustained by the vital interplay between two opposing forces. Chinese philosophy refers to these forces as yin and yang. (They have also been called Shiva and Shakti in other traditions, or the divine feminine and divine masculine.) It is the union of these polarising energies that offers us wholeness and balance, and the synergy of these opposite but complementary forces is dependent on a delicate balance: if the pendulum swings too much in one direction, the harmony of our world is compromised.

At the micro level, our individual wholeness is affected by the internal relationship between these energies. The qualities of yin can include birthing, mothering, relaxation, grace, psychic connection, and gentleness; and being nurturing, nourishing, trusting, grounding, receptive, intuitive, creative, sensitive, slow and soft. Yin is our connection to spirit, the energy of the moon and the silent strength of night, and these qualities are often associated with the right hemisphere of our brain. Yang qualities, by contrast, can include power, courage, leadership, protection, strength and speed; and being action-oriented. Yang is the heat of the sun and the active energy of the day, and the left hemisphere of our brain is often correlated with the qualities of yang.

Tipping the balance

The terms 'masculine' and 'feminine' are heavily loaded words that can trigger us as a result of years of cultural conditioning around what it supposedly means to be male or female. This conditioning has distorted the balance of our natural qualities – the yin and yang in our world and within ourselves. Regardless of how we self-identify on a gendered spectrum, these dual energies coexist in our being, irrespective of our biological sex. When yin and yang are balanced and in harmony, we transcend their duality and can be flexible in using whatever qualities are needed in any given moment to support our well-being.

But when these qualities are out of balance and one force becomes more dominant, we experience disharmony. Moreover, when one of these energies is pushed to extremes without the complementary balance of the opposing force, yin can manifest as submissive, lacking boundaries and passive, while yang can be overly ambitious, rigid, aggressive and controlling. We can see the imbalance of these forces in the business, economic, educational and political structures of our modern world. Today's world is governed by the extreme qualities of yang, which are often revered as superior and more desirable. We are missing the equitable presence of yin energies, and as a result we have disturbance, disharmony and possible disintegration at the macro and micro levels. But we are each being called to reimagine a world where we can live, learn, work and play in a way that honours the natural rhythms, cycles and energies that reside within each of us.

Bringing yin and yang together

Our natural rhythm is a harmonious dance between yin and yang, but we have altered this organic equilibrium to try to fit into current world systems. As women, we have been pushed to live a life dominated by yang energy. Our innate yin qualities have been seen as weaker and not as valuable in the global economy. In an effort to try to fit into this structure, we have suppressed our cyclical nature and our yin qualities and allowed yang to take centre stage. The same is true for men. The conditioned concept of masculinity has asked men to suppress and deny their intrinsic yin qualities. This has caused much harm and suffering to both sexes, to our relationships with each other, and to how we connect to the planet.

Both energies are needed in right relationship, pulsing together to complement each other. Living out of sync with our natural qualities pushes us to the brink of collapse. The cumulative effects of our imbalanced lifestyle impact our well-being at all levels: physical, energetic, mental, emotional and spiritual. Many of us may be unaware of how this is affecting us, but as we cross the threshold into our forties and beyond, it starts to become more obvious. Every system in the body relies on equilibrium, and when we compound this with the biological changes happening at midlife, the effects can be overwhelming. Healing at all levels of our being is needed to help us come back to our true self. In midlife, we are called to reflect on our past, nurse old wounds and embody the wisdom gained as we explore our present to discover how we can create a future life that is aligned with how we want to be in the world.

The Age of Aquarius

While I acknowledge that not all readers of this book will be familiar with or value astrology, I believe that the imbalance between yin and yang that we are experiencing on the macro scale can be understood from an astrological point of view in the context of the Age of Pisces. This is the astrological age we have been experiencing for the last 2,000 years or so. Astrological ages reflect major shifts and changes in our cultural, societal and political landscape, and the Age of Pisces has been marked by the rise in Christianity, globalisation and a patriarchal society. The earth is now on the threshold of entering into a new age – the Age of Aquarius.

Jean Shinoda Bolen, a psychiatrist, activist and author, describes this time as *liminal time*.[6] She says that 'liminal' defines the time in between *what was* and *what is next*. This in-between phase can feel like a time of great ambiguity, loss and suffering, but it is also a remarkable opportunity for growth, learning and rebirth. Astrologers predict that the Age of Aquarius can be an age of renewal, in which a more egalitarian society can be created as women and men share power, working together more harmoniously. But this positive transition can only arise if the seeds of transformation are now planted. After the intensity of the last few years of the global pandemic, many of us have felt in our bones that great change is coming. As we witnessed the undoing of so many of our systems and structures, we may intuitively know that it is time for deep contemplation on how we currently live our lives collectively.

The liminal time of midlife

The macro transition between the astrological ages is not unlike what is happening to us as we approach the threshold of midlife. As we move out of our thirties and into our forties, fifties and beyond, we may experience a sense of liminal time. At midlife, we leave behind an old version of ourselves and enter an in-between space where we are discovering who we are becoming. Shinoda Bolen says this is a critical juncture, when we come to know ourselves better and find out how we can be more useful in the world.[7]

Unfortunately, the Western culture that many of us have been born into, and which developed during the Age of Pisces, would have us believe that as we move into midlife and lose our reproductive value, we emerge onto a scrapheap like dilapidated cars that have lost their worth. Moreover, with so much of a woman's self-worth being constructed on societal images of youthful beauty, we can be forgiven for thinking we *do* actually belong on the scrapheap. We must remember, however, that the new culture we can cocreate in the next phase of the earth depends on what ideas we plant now.

The harmonising of yin and yang is crucial for tipping humanity towards a more egalitarian future, and the wisdom of women has never been more needed. As we step into our power, we can lift and support men. Many people would say it is a difficult time to be a man. Women are conditioned to expect men to be super masculine and excessively yang. We can find ourselves feeling insecure when men show vulnerability and more sensitive qualities. Yet when we step fully into our power, we are secure in ourselves and we can hold the space to allow men to feel safer in opening up to their innate yin qualities. When women are whole and authentic, we give men permission to be their fullest and most whole self, and it is healing for both biological sexes. We are ancestors in training, and the work we do now with the rest of our lives will determine how we hand over the earth to our children's children and their children. Becoming conscious stewards of the earth, we can strive to play our part wisely and contribute positively to sowing the seeds of safety, wholeness, peace and harmony for future generations.

The feminine archetypes

Carl Jung, a Swiss psychologist and psychiatrist, developed the concept of archetypes to help us better understand our social roles and patterns. From an evolutionary perspective, archetypes evolved to support humans living together in tribes and communities.

An archetype describes the force behind our behaviours and includes particular character traits, motivations and patterns that are common across all our cultures, stories, myths and legends.

In the 1980s, Shinoda Bolen took the work of Carl Jung and pioneered the development of the seven female archetypes in her book *Goddesses in Every-woman*.[8] Each of us can embody the energy of all seven of these archetypes, although we may feel that one resonates more strongly with us or that we are yet to tap into a particular archetype within us. Over the course of our lives, our relationship with the energies of the archetypes might shift and change. And given that we are cyclical beings, we might find that we lean into a certain archetypal energy at particular points during our menstrual cycle and different seasons of our lives.

Working with archetypal patterns allows us to understand our own unique strengths and the gifts that we came to offer the world. Archetypes can also reveal to us innate traits that we may be suppressing in an effort to fit into our family or wider society. With this awareness, we can work to break down patterns that no longer serve us and consciously activate qualities that may be hidden within us.

The archetypes also help us to see that we are made up of both light and dark. By becoming acquainted with our shadow side, we start to understand how this part of us might cause difficulties and tensions in our relationships with others. Furthermore, leaning into one archetype too heavily might restrict the presence of other archetypes within us. By becoming more whole and balanced, we allow space for all of these archetypal energies to flow within us and radiate outwards. This helps to expand our possibilities, enabling us to become a fuller expression of who we truly are and to access the courage to carry out what we came here to do.

The Seven Feminine Archetypes[9]

The Maiden: She represents the daughter, innocent and pure. She also embodies beauty, youth and hopefulness. This is the energy of playfulness, curiosity, imagination and dreams. In folklore, the maiden can fall under spells and is at risk of manipulation. The maiden is represented in Greek mythology by the goddess Persephone, who was kidnapped by her uncle Hades, and in Roman mythology by the goddess Proserpina, who was abducted by Pluto. In these stories, the kidnapping of the maiden can symbolise the transition from innocence to experience.

The Mother: She is loving and maternal, whether she has her own children or not. She is a natural caregiver, who nurtures and nourishes others and is the keeper of the hearth or home. This is the energy of love, selflessness, generosity, support and service to others. She symbolises the earth and the harvest. The mother is a creator, who can birth something into being. She carries a lot of responsibilities, and others are dependent on her. Her energy can be prone to burnout from overgiving. She is represented by the Greek goddess

Demeter and the Roman goddess Ceres – both goddesses of the harvest.

The Wild Woman: She is intuitive and expressive. She feels things deeply and is a truth teller. The wild woman is a warrior or a huntress. Independent and autonomous, she questions the status quo and is a catalyst for change, ready to take action. This is the energy of bravery, courage and fearlessness. She represents all that is wild and natural. Her energy can manifest as rage and anger at the current structures, and she is here to challenge and to encourage change and transformation. She is represented by the Greek goddess Artemis and the Roman goddess Diana – the goddesses of the natural world and the moon.

The Sage: She embodies the lived experience of truth, knowledge and wisdom. She is a guide, a healer, a knower and a seer. She is spiritual and is deeply connected to the truth and the cycles of life. This is the energy of the wise woman – or the elders and ancestors. She is intuitive, with an inner power and strength. She inspires others to connect to their wisdom and truth. In mythology, she is the Greek goddess Athena and the Roman goddess Minerva – the goddesses of wisdom.

The Mystic: She is deeply spiritual and connected to the universe. She feels things intensely and is very intuitive. She is introverted and enjoys a rich inner life. She craves solitude and introspection. This is the energy of inner peace, divinity and tranquillity. She is here to guide us inwards to find the spiritual meaning in our lives. The mystic is represented by the Greek goddess Hestia and the Roman goddess Vesta – the goddesses of the temple and peacekeepers.

The Queen: She is confident, committed and loyal. She is motivated to create meaningful alliances. This is the energy of brave leadership and power. The queen has an inner fire, and she attracts what she wants. She is here to lead and empower. She is represented by the Greek goddess Hera and the Roman goddess Juno.

The Lover: She is creative, sensual and loving. She enjoys pleasure and beauty. This is the energy of creativity, sensuality and sexuality. She is the overarching energy of love. She is here to encourage us to create, to take beauty and pleasure in the world, and to expand our circle of love. The lover symbolises connection, intimacy, relationships and togetherness. She is represented by the Greek goddess Aphrodite and the Roman goddess Venus – associated with love, passion, desire and beauty.

PRACTICE: Finding your primary archetype[10]

Take a moment to consider the list of seven feminine archetypes. You may want to have a notebook and pen to use as you reflect on:

- Which archetype resonates with you most?
- Which archetypal energy do you identify with the least?
- Which archetypal energy would you like to bring more of into your way of being in the world?
- At times in your life, have you had to repress one of these archetypes?
- In your life now, which qualities have you been afraid to demonstrate?
- What qualities have you felt you should demonstrate instead?
- What are you afraid will happen if you fully embrace all parts of your nature?

How do we navigate this quest?

During this liminal time, we need tools to navigate this inner experience of getting to know ourselves better. The chapters that follow in this book offer some practices that can be used to support our journey. We also need guides, mentors and role models. The Sufi poet Rumi advised that when setting out on a journey we should not seek advice from those who have never left home.[11] Instead, we can seek out the wisdom of others who have crossed the threshold and are activating their power and living their purpose. We can look out for possible mentors and teachers that come into our life to enthuse us and show us the way. We need to hear the stories of those who are courageously living in a way that inspires us to rethink how we live our own lives. We can be open to finding new role models who are expressing themselves authentically. They may be living a life in a way that is different to the old status quo, without harming others. They are natural leaders who can motivate us to question everything we have been taught to accept and believe. From their stories, we can find strength and courage to transform how we live our own lives.

CASE STUDY: Danielle and her wife Maria underwent many rounds of IVF until they happily found themselves expecting their first child. Excited to prepare for their new baby, they went shopping for their first baby clothes. As they walked through the shopping centre hand in hand, enjoying this special time, a stranger approached them and verbally abused them with homophobic comments. Instantly, Maria dropped Danielle's hand. She was deeply hurt by his comments and felt ashamed. Her protective instinct was to hide their relationship. Danielle remained calm and asked Maria to hold hands again. She said it was important that they fully accept themselves and express their commitment to each other, despite the negative bias that

still exists in the world towards same-sex
relationships. Danielle believed strongly that
they could only bring a child into the world
when they had fully accepted who they were,
as they needed to be able to demonstrate
and impart that to their child. This has been
their mantra ever since – fully embracing who
they are so that they can teach their children
self-acceptance. Our children are constantly
watching us, mirroring us. If we deny the
fullest expression of who we are, we teach our
children to do the same.

The world needs our wisdom

We need unity to support each other, to welcome each
other, to show each other compassion and forgiveness,
and to offer each other a sense of belonging. We are all
here in this world together. Each of us belongs on this
planet and has a right to be here. The archetypal energy
of the mother or caregiver that is within us all (regardless of whether we have children or not) has been a
guiding light in compassionate conversation, diplomacy
and negotiation since the first families began. This is
one of the many wise qualities of leadership that we can
offer the world. We can actively listen, without judgement, to voices that are different, and try to understand
the motivations that influence and inform.

This is how we create a more peaceful, unified world, rather than by shutting people out. Can we show more compassion and understanding to ourselves and others, acknowledging that we don't always know everything? We are each a work in progress, not a static, complete and finished product. Our nature is dynamic and transient, and we are each here to learn, grow and evolve. There are many opportunities for learning on our path. We don't always grab them because we are afraid to try and afraid to fail. If we let fear hold us back, we limit ourselves and push opportunities away. By tapping into the energy of both our wild and wise feminine archetypes, we can gain more confidence and courage to rise up, and we can trust what is in our hearts so that we can try to begin sharing our gifts with the world. By fully embracing our yin qualities and the energies of all seven of the feminine archetypes, we gain clarity, wisdom and courage to offer new ways of communicating, leading, collaborating, serving and supporting each other and our planet.

PRACTICE: Tapping to awaken your dormant energies

This is a practice you can use to awaken the energy or archetypal qualities that you want to reclaim, and also to let go of what you no longer need. Start standing tall with the feet a little wider than your hips. Bring your hands to the top of your head. Consider the qualities you want to reawaken.

With both hands, begin to tap the crown of your head with your fingertips, and then move down the side of your head and the back of your head.

As you tap, visualise that you are awakening these dormant energies within you. Continue to tap down your forehead, temples, cheeks, jaw, neck and throat. Then, making the hands into fists, begin to tap across the chest and the collar bones. Make the hands flatter as you tap the side ribs, the front of the hips, the lower back, the back of the hips and the buttocks. Tap down both arms. Then, bending the knees, begin to tap down the front of the thighs, the backs of the thighs, the shins and the calves, all the way to the feet. Curl up slowly, back to standing.

Now begin to consider all the old habits, patterns or shadow qualities that no longer serve you. Bring the hands back to the top of the head and brush down the body, with the intention that you are brushing off what you want to let go of. Brush or sweep the hands from the crown, down the sides of the head, down the face, the neck and the shoulders. Brush down the chest, the belly, the hips, the lower back and the buttocks. Then brush down both arms. Bending the knees again, begin to brush down the front and back of the legs, all the way to the feet. Sense that you are not only brushing off the qualities that you want to release, but also the heavy expectations and burdens of others. Allow them to be released to the earth. Coming back up to standing, take a deep breath in through the nose and a deep exhale through the mouth. Notice how you feel. Use this practice any time you need to feel lighter and more yourself.

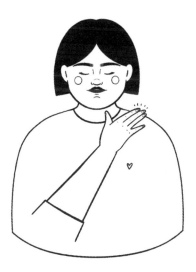

Pearls of wisdom

- Our needs matter.
- When our tank is full, we can give to others.
- The wisdom of women is needed to transform our world.
- It is our responsibility to be change-makers.
- We feel the call of our soul to be impactful during the transition to midlife.

○ We are called on a quest to journey inwards and retrieve our power.

○ It is time to take off our mask and step into our authenticity.

○ Doing this work requires us to come back to wholeness, to live in rhythm, and to balance our energies.

○ Remember, we can access the energy of the seven feminine archetypes to support us on this journey.

CHAPTER TWO

The Age of Wisdom

*"A self that goes on changing
is a self that goes on living."*

VIRGINIA WOOLF

Since I was young, I have always been intrigued by stories of people who seemed to discover their gifts later in life – like Vera Wang, who started designing wedding dresses at 40 years of age, or Julia Child, who published her first cookbook at 49 years of age. And just recently, Angela Álvarez started her recording career at 90 years of age, winning best new Latin artist award at the Grammy Awards when she was 95 years old. In a youth-obsessed culture, these women are not only inspiring, but serve to remind us that it is okay not to have everything figured out yet. There is time to get to know ourselves and bring something to the world later in life. Western culture, however, doesn't always encourage us to think this way. Our society does not see the value of ageing as a time to assimilate and embody wisdom, and so we don't honour the wisdom of our elders.

Many of us have been conditioned through aggressive marketing campaigns to try to prevent the natural ageing process. Our propensity for fear and shame at the visible signs of ageing is worth a lot of money to the companies that sell us a promise of eternal youth – the global anti-ageing market is worth over $45 billion.[1] Our rejection of ageing appears to stem from a deeply ingrained fear of death in our psyche. We try to resist death by clinging to youth and going to war against the physical signs of ageing. Youthfulness is applauded as beautiful and worthy, with the result that those of us who dare to age find our self-worth diminishing in a world that tells us we should remain young. The passage into midlife sees our inner maiden flourish into a wilder, wiser woman. If we embrace the energies of these archetypes, we will see a great shift in the world. But sadly, many women feel the desire to hide these qualities in an anti-ageing culture. We suppress our inner wise woman to try to fit in and conform.

Can we accept that change is inevitable?

The anti-ageing narrative is anti-life and anti-growth. When we start to accept impermanence and death as inescapable parts of the cycle of life, we gain immense freedom, clarity and perspective to truly live. To age is to grow, and everything that is living must age. Ageing gives us the opportunity to learn, change, evolve and gain the perspective, clarity and wisdom that only comes with a life fully lived. This is something to be celebrated, embraced and honoured. And as we know, it is a privilege denied to many people who died before they reached this stage of life.

Is it time for a new vision?

Despite what the marketeers want us to believe, the truth is that we cannot beat ageing or escape death. Denying the natural stages of life is futile. Moreover, it is damaging to ourselves. We lose connection with our natural rhythms and damage our well-being. We are exhausted and experience epidemic levels of illness and burnout trying to conform to a system not designed with our wholeness in mind.

But we have the power to shift our reality. We can create a radical new paradigm that values personal growth and the balance of yin and yang, and that ritualises the cycles of life. This transformation begins with us. It can only happen when each of us realises that we have something wise and sacred to contribute. Midlife often gives us the opportunity to fully embrace all that we are and all that we can be. If we can intentionally lean into the flow of this liminal time, we can find more fulfilment. But if we push against the rhythm of this rite of passage, then we will suffer.

The crisis of midlife

The term 'midlife crisis' was coined by Jung to describe the journey we pursue to find purpose and meaning in the second half of life.[2] Jung believed that people experience crisis when they have not been true to themselves or when they live in an inauthentic way that is out of alignment with who they really are. He suggested that the quest of midlife is to reconnect with our uniqueness and individuality and to follow the path intended for us by nature. Jung's treatment for a midlife crisis involved asking patients to tune into their imagination and creativity and to rediscover hidden parts of themselves, such as the passions and interests they had in adolescence. From the Jungian perspective, midlife is a chance to return to ourselves, getting to know ourselves in a deeper way and unearthing meaning in our lives.

Interestingly, the word 'crisis' has its origins in the Greek *krisis*, which means 'a critical turning point or decision'. Similarly, the word crisis is interpreted in Chinese as a 'change point'. Midlife is a significant turning point in our lives. Up until this time, typically we have been in striving mode – focused on the pursuit of educational achievements, meeting a partner, building our families and following a hierarchical career path to accumulate material goods. As strivers, we allow our value and worth to be measured by our accomplishments and financial success. But Professor Arthur Brooks of Harvard says that this linear path leaves us unfulfilled, as we suffer the 'striver's curse', finding that attaining our material desires and achievements does not provide the meaning that we need in our lives.[3]

Thinking back to Maslow's work, we can see that although material things make life more comfortable, they only help us to fulfil our lower level in the hierarchy of needs.[4] Focusing solely on our material desires, and ignoring our higher-level needs for safety, love, self-actualisation, transcendence and spiritual connection, does not give us more contentment. In fact, the law of diminishing returns sets in, and no matter how much more personal wealth and material goods we accumulate, our lives will lack meaning and purpose until we begin to address our desire for love, connection and the highest human potential.

The five universal elements

The principles of *Ayurveda*, the Indian science of life, can help us to understand ourselves better and make sense of the shifts and changes during midlife. In Sanskrit, *ayur* means life and *veda* means knowledge. Yoga is one well-known practice that is derived from Ayurveda. According to Ayurveda, the universe is made up of five elements: ether (or space), air, earth, fire and water. Crucially, each element is needed to give us life and sustain us.

Just like the universe, each of us is made up of a combination of these elements, and some of us will have more of one element than others. The unique combination of elements that we have will form our natural constitution and influence the qualities of our mind, body and spirit. Jennifer Freed, a psychologist and astrologer, says that when we know our personal map of these elements we can take care of ourselves better and design our best life, which is one that allows us to fully express our unique gifts.[5] The science of Ayurveda offers us a way to explore our personal map of these elements by working with our *doshas*. A dosha is a combination of two universal elements that come together to make up a predominant force within us. This force will have a tendency to go out of balance if we don't consciously live in a way that supports our personal make-up.

The three doshas

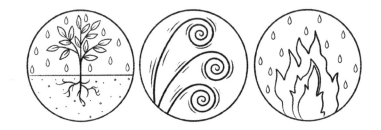

There are three primary doshas called *kapha*, *pitta* and *vata*. Each of us will have a dosha or a combination of doshas that can go out of balance. When this happens, we must use opposing elements to bring more harmony and balance into our life. Furthermore, according to Ayurveda, each stage of life is governed by a predominant dosha that must be considered to restore balance at that time of our life. Let's look at the qualities of each dosha and the stage of life that it represents.

Kapha dosha: The primary elements of kapha are earth and water. The kapha stage of life is from birth to puberty. It sustains our growth and development during these years. Some of the qualities of kapha are coolness, heaviness, density, slowness, stability, empathy, wisdom, support, nourishment and care. When kapha goes out of balance, we can experience inertia, lethargy, fatigue and lack of motivation.

Pitta dosha: The primary elements of pitta are fire and water. Pitta is responsible for metabolism, digestion and transformation in the body. The pitta stage of life is from puberty to late forties or early fifties. This stage of life is about striving, learning, taking action and assimilating all of our experiences. It is also the time of life where we are most driven to achieve. Some of the qualities of pitta include warmth, oiliness, sharpness, lightness, liquidness and fluidity. It is associated with strength, action, purpose, goals and tasks. Excess pitta in our system can cause excessive heat, anger, rage, impatience, conflict and inflammation.

Vata dosha: The primary elements of vata are air and ether. Like the wind, vata is responsible for all movement and transportation within the body and for the breath. Some of the qualities of vata include lightness, coolness, dryness, spaciousness, creativity and flexibility. The vata stage of life relates to midlife and beyond. During this stage, everything in the body is becoming drier. We can sense this dryness in our skin, in the fluid in our joints, in loss of hair pigment and in brittle hair. Our eye health and cognitive abilities may also be affected. When we have excess vata, we can be easily distracted, anxious, forgetful and restless. But importantly, vata also offers us the chance to expand our consciousness and spiritual growth.

How to transition smoothly to the Age of Vata

At every stage of life, our well-being is optimised when we live in a way that brings our three doshas into balance and harmony. At the macro level, the cycle of midlife brings more vata to manage. But within this context, we will have our own individual constitution of the elements, established at birth and defining our predisposed tendency for imbalance. Knowing our individual dosha can be empowering. With this knowledge, we can be aware of the signs that we are out of balance and consciously work with the opposite elements to find more balance in our life.

For example, we can tame excess pitta with earth and water (kapha). We ground vata with earth and water (kapha). We get ourselves out of the mud (kapha) with action (pitta) and more uplifting movement (vata). Having this knowledge, we can lean into appropriate food choices, movement practices, self-care and relaxation tools that give us more of the elements we are lacking to bring us back into equanimity. Tools that work for one may not work for all. It is important to have this self-knowledge so we can prevent the accumulation of imbalances with tailored approaches that suit us personally.

PRACTICE: Find your dosha

This is a practice to help you discover which dosha is most likely to go out of balance for you.[6] Read the following questionnaire and select the responses that best describe

you. Add up your responses for each column of vata, pitta
and kapha. The column with the highest score is your
predominant dosha and the one that is most likely to go
out of balance. It is possible to score high on two doshas,
which means you have a propensity for imbalance in both
of these doshas.

THE DOSHA QUESTIONNAIRE

PHYSICAL FEATURES	VATA	PITTA	KAPHA
BODY FRAME	Thin, bones are prominent, rarely gains weight	Medium build, can gain and lose weight easily	Large; round; gains weight easily and finds it difficult to lose it
HEIGHT	Tall or short	Medium height	Short to medium
SKIN	Normal to dry; cool; rough; thin; prone to dry, dull and wrinkly skin – has cold hands and feet	Normal to oily; soft; reddish freckles; sensitive; warm; skin can be prone to inflammation and irritation	Normal to oily; soft; cool; wet; thick; pale; prone to itchy skin and fungal infections

	VATA	PITTA	KAPHA
SWEAT	Minimal sweat and odour	Sweats profusely and has a medium body odour	Sweats moderately except when working hard; has a strong body odour
HAIR	Rough, dry, thin, wavy, dark, knotted, brittle hair; gets split ends easily	Normal, straight, thin, brownish, blonde or red hair; can have early greying and balding	Oily, lustrous, thick, curly hair, with the colour being on the darker side
EYES	Small, dry and sleepy eyes; eyes tend to blink a lot	Medium-sized – sharp, search-ing and shiny eyes; eyes tend to get reddish often	Big, calm, attractive and smiling eyes, with thick eye lashes
TONGUE	Dry, pale and smaller, with black spots	Reddish and medium	Bigger; fuller; whitish; easily develops a white coating
LIPS AND TEETH	Thin, dry lips that can get cracked easily; teeth may be uneven, crook-ed, irregular in shape and/or size, requiring continual attention	Medium-sized, red, moist, soft lips with upper lip being darker than lower; teeth are medium sized; can suffer with cavities	Large, thick, full and smooth lips; teeth are aligned well and tend not to require a very high level of care
HIPS	Small; slim	Medium	Large

	VATA	PITTA	KAPHA
NAILS	Dry; rough; flaky; weak; irregular shape	Pink and soft, with a nice shape	Wide and whitish, but thick and smooth
ACTIVITIES			
WALK AND TALK	Fast	Moderate	Slow and steady
SLEEP	Light and disturbed; wakes up easily in the morning; can suffer from insomnia	Moderate and regular sleep; can go back to sleep easily	Deep and heavy sleep; difficult to wake up in the morning
APPETITE	Irregular; tends to pick at food	Strong appetite – always hungry! Gets angry if not able to eat on time	Steady and enjoys a big plate when it arrives; eats for comfort and taste
DIGESTION AND BOWELS	Can be irregular, constipated, bloated and gassy	Regular, but can suffer from acidity, heartburn and loose stools	Sluggish, lethargic and bulky stools
PERSONAL ATTRIBUTES	Creative; imaginative; visionary	Organised; passionate; perfectionist; confident	Reliable; loyal; hardworking; kind

	VATA	PITTA	KAPHA
WEATHER INDICATION	Enjoys the summer heat and is uncomfortable during the cold season	Dislikes heat, but enjoys a cool climate	Mostly comfortable, but prefers the summer and spring and dislikes damp; enjoys sunshine over shade

MENTAL AND EMOTIONAL ATTRIBUTES

	VATA	PITTA	KAPHA
EMOTIONAL NATURE	Worries a lot; often feels nervous and anxious	Easily irritated, angry and impatient	Loving and caring; it takes a lot to elicit anger
MIND ON PERFORMING ACTIONS	Overthinks	Quick implementation	Slow; has a tendency to procrastinate
MEMORY	Quick to learn and quick to forget; has a good short-term memory	Takes an average time to learn; good overall memory	Slow to learn, but remembers for a long time; long-term memory is good
MENTAL ACTIVITY	Mind tends to get restless easily; insecure and anxious; overthinks	Mind gets impatient and aggressive easily; jealous; angry	Mostly cool and calm; rarely gets ruffled

FOR WOMEN ONLY			
	VATA	PITTA	KAPHA
MENSTRUAL CYCLE	Irregular; clots; intense cramps; dark colour; scanty flow; mild PMS with tearfulness	Regular; heavy; bleeds for a long time; bright red; medium cramps; bad PMS with irritability	Regular, easy periods; dull cramps; water retention; mild PMS
MENOPAUSE SIGNS	Dryness; memory loss; difficulty in concentrating and sleeping; anxiety; possible bone loss	Experiences excess heat; skin imbalances; angry and irritable; possible heart irregularities	Weight gain; heaviness; low mood or depression; possible increased cholesterol

The doshas and midlife

As we know, midlife is governed by vata dosha. It is a time when our system is releasing excess heat (pitta) to allow for more lightness and space for expansion (vata). During midlife, we can consciously support ourselves to have a smoother release of this built-up pitta, while balancing the increased vata that is part of the natural ageing process, by embracing the qualities of kapha. Including more kapha in our lives can help us to manage the symptoms of excess pitta and increasing vata. We can do this by working with the elements of water and earth that make up kapha. Through grounding, slow and cooling movement practices, we can let go of the heat and feel more anchored in the midst of a lot of vata. We can eat kapha foods like soups and stews to ground vata. We can walk barefoot in nature to feel grounded or bathe in water to cool down.

It must be emphasised that the natural changes in the elements that happen during midlife are not all negative. The expansiveness of vata gives us huge potential for emotional, spiritual and creative growth. If we resist this change by clinging to a past image of ourselves, we may miss these possibilities for growth. With the wisdom of acceptance, we can get curious and playful about how this stage of life can lead to great transformation and bring about greater meaning.

What is happening to our hormones?

As we reach our forties and prepare for transition from the pitta into the vata stage of life, we are releasing the accumulation of heat (pitta) and gaining more qualities of vata. This maps the biological changes in the endocrine system that occur at this time of life. The endocrine system, controlled by the brain, governs the production and release of hormones in the body. We cannot talk about midlife without mentioning hormones, as to varying degrees both biological females and biological males will experience significant neurochemical and hormonal changes during the transition to midlife.

Biological male andropause

Although less well known, men too experience endocrine changes as they transition into midlife. 'Andropause' is the medical term given to the declining levels of testosterone in the male biological body. Anywhere from 30 to 40 years of age, testosterone begins to decline by about 2 per cent per year. Although these hormonal changes in males happen at a much slower pace than in females, pitta is releasing and vata is increasing, so symptoms can be similar and just as significant. There can be adverse cardiovascular effects, declining bone density, decreased libido, erectile dysfunction, decreased muscle strength, increased irritability, low mood, and a risk of depression and anxiety.

Female perimenopause and menopause

The biological female's journey to midlife includes *perimenopause* and *menopause*. Perimenopause is the time leading up to the cessation of the menstrual cycle and it begins most commonly from our mid-forties. Indeed, women from 45 years of age are assumed to be perimenopausal by the medical profession.[7] During perimenopause, the level of the sex hormones oestrogen and progesterone are fluctuating and declining in the body and our periods may be irregular. A woman is medically defined as being menopausal one year after her last period, signalling the end of her reproductive life. The average age of menopause in the Western world is 51 years of age.[8] However, 1 in 100 women experience premature menopause before 40 years of age and 1 in 1,000 before the age of 30.[9] Some women experience menopause naturally, while others will go through menopause as the result of medical or surgical treatment.

Symptoms of the female hormonal waves

The hormonal waves in midlife reflect the shifting doshas, and as many of us will have already noticed, each of us may experience the symptoms differently. The releasing heat of pitta can manifest as hot flushes, night sweats, heavier menstruation, and cardiovascular issues. We can also experience fiery emotions, such as irritability, anger and rage. As pitta releases, the fire of the metabolism also slows down and our bodies change shape and gain weight. As we accumulate more vata in our system, we feel less juicy in our body, as everything is becoming drier, like the quality of air. This can commonly manifest as aches and pains in the joints, dry skin and hair loss. Our bone density declines at a rate of 1 per cent per year, putting us at a higher risk of osteoporosis and associated fractures. We might also experience changes in the tissues of the vulva, vagina, urethra and bladder, resulting in prolapses and incontinence, vaginal dryness or irritation, a changing libido and painful sex. Other symptoms can include anxiety, low mood, brain fog, loss of confidence and deteriorating concentration, and in some severe cases women can experience personality disintegration.

Getting the right support

For some of us, the hormonal decline is a rapid crash. This can be damaging to our physical and mental health if we are not prepared and educated about the sudden onset of symptoms and about what help is available. Having a sense of awareness of the role of our sex hormones and the effect their decline has on us allows us to prepare for the changes. Knowledge is power and can encourage a smoother transition to this stage of life.

Whilst a quarter of women will journey through menopause relatively unscathed, for many of us the symptoms may feel overwhelming, and we may require medical advice.[10] What works for one person will not work for another, so it is best to seek out an individual, tailored approach to holistic support and treatment options for symptoms, perhaps including hormone replacement therapy (HRT), to manage symptoms in a way that is right for our own well-being.

Interestingly, and while taking care not to downplay the experiences of many women, significant research shows that the values in our culture can affect our meno-pause experiences. In societies where age is more revered and older women are seen as wiser, women may experience menopausal symptoms as significantly less challenging.[11] In Japan, where the very word for menopause, *konenki*, means renewal, season and energy – women report less severe symptoms.[12] In the Middle East, Asia and among First Nations people, a woman can find she is more respected in her community when she enters menopause because her wisdom is acknowledged. By contrast, in societies that are anti-ageing, women may experience more disturbing symptoms. If we can shift the collective culture to respect the natural balance of yin and yang and our female rhythms, and honour the wisdom that comes from transitioning to midlife, then we might see a change in the quality of life for millions of perimenopausal and menopausal women.

Attuning to our female rhythms

As biological females, we have been experiencing the rise and fall of hormonal changes throughout our monthly cycles since puberty. Perhaps many of us have lived this experience without much awareness. Menstrual cycle awareness (MCA) is a process of becoming more conscious of our monthly cycle and attuning to our natural rhythms. It is critical for helping us to under-stand the biological rhythm that impacts our physical bodies, emotions, mindset and energy, and our intuitive connection during the cyclical waves of our hormones. When we are aware of these rhythms, we can make informed choices to adjust how we live to be more in sync with this cycle, helping us to feel more resourced, balanced and harmonious.

PRACTICE: Menstrual cycle awareness

The process of MCA is very simple. It can involve tracking our monthly cycle with technology or in a diary and noting changes in the physical body, emotions or undulating moods, energy levels, libido, sensitivity to others, etc. As we tune into our cycle, we gain more clarity on how our needs (physically, energetically, mentally, emotionally and spiritually) shift and change as our hormones fluctuate during the month. With this knowledge, we can adapt our lifestyle and personal commitments to match what we need at different times during the month.

It is never too late to develop this awareness, and in fact it is particularly useful to help us become aware of the hormonal waves of midlife. It can be done whether you have a menstrual cycle or not. Leaning into menstrual cycle awareness during our transition to midlife can help us to identify any emerging symptoms of our hormonal decline. Without this information, we might not connect the dots of our experience with hormonal changes. This could cause us to miss out on critical advice and treatment options that might really benefit us and, in some cases, might actually save us.

Is there a purpose behind the hormonal changes?

The hormonal changes can be radical and bring a lot of uncertainty, but they do pave the way for us to transform, emerge and step into our wise power. For example, when oestrogen decreases in our bodies, it can have a positive effect in helping us connect with our authentic truth. We become less interested in people pleasing, because we are no longer concerned with reproducing. We may feel more empowered as natural leaders, something that we may have been more reluctant about before, out of fear of what others would think of us. Considering the hormonal changes as facilitators of personal growth can help us to embrace this transition with less trepidation. Knowing what the purpose of change is and the gifts that it can bring us, we can begin to see how the transition might actually serve us. With the right knowledge and support, we don't have to suffer. Instead, we can use this time for inner growth and positive transformation.

CASE STUDY: At 41 years of age, Samantha was diagnosed with endometriosis, a painful condition in which tissue that normally lines the uterus grows outside the uterus. The doctors recommended a full hysterectomy, removing her uterus and both ovaries. Her goal, when she came to me for yoga therapy post-surgery, was to use yoga to help her physically recover from the surgery and regain her core strength. Before surgery, she was very active, hiking and running most days. During our sessions, she revealed to me that she was experiencing very low moods and finding it hard to get out of bed some days.

Now she felt anxious and paranoid. Her surgery had induced menopause without the natural lead-up of perimenopause. She was surprised and unprepared for the rapid crash of hormones associated with a surgical menopause. Because of her age, she had not given much thought to the menopause, and she had not considered that her low mood might be a result of her shift in hormones. After her surgery, the hospital had given Samantha a prescription for HRT but no other information around the symptoms of menopause. I advised her to urgently make an appointment with a doctor to talk about her low mood and get advice on the best medication to support her. Thankfully, she found a female doctor with more specialist training in menopause. She was prescribed a different combination of HRT and medication to relieve her anxiety. As her body healed from surgery, she made a conscious effort to be more active outdoors again and found this helped her to feel more like herself. Over the next few months, she found her mood was up and down, but empowered with an understanding of the transition she was experiencing, Samantha found she could be kinder and more patient with herself.

Shifting our focus inwards

All too often, I hear stories from older clients who have come through the perimenopause and menopausal years and who say they went through 10 years of hell without understanding what was going on with their hormones. In the past, women were silent about the physical symptoms of this time of life. They made this journey without any support, feeling alone and like they were losing their mind.

Fortunately, the voices of women are now rising up to share their experiences, and a medical community, driven largely by female practitioners who themselves realised the dearth of support during their own transition, is creating more awareness and education around the symptoms. Open conversation and awareness represent a great leap forward for women's health and mental well-being during this time of life. But we also need to shift the cultural anti-ageing narrative to value the wisdom of women as we age. There is still a greater emphasis on what we lose during midlife rather than what we gain, creating a sense of fear and dread about this time of life and compounding the stress around what is already a challenging time. And as we have seen, many of our sisters who live in cultures that value ageing, and who therefore feel an increased social standing as they age, often experience less difficult symptoms.

We cannot change society overnight, but we can make a shift within ourselves. If we only focus on the exterior, we overlook the inner landscape. We each have a profound inner potential, but we inhibit ourselves through self-criticism, shame, guilt, lack of self-worth, embarrassment, fear, and worry about what others will think. An amazing thing happens during midlife: if we stop objectifying ourselves for our exterior ageing appearance, we start to remember that we are much more than our physical bodies and we shift our focus inwards.

This is the most beautiful time in our life for self-enquiry. By exploring our interior, we get to know ourselves better. We begin to notice how things feel rather than how they look. This simple shift inwards can have a profound effect on our sense of self. Through the lens of awareness, we can develop a deeper relationship with ourselves, which ripples out into how we relate to others in the world. As we move inwards on a journey of self-study, we become conscious of the many layers of our being. We start to see a glimpse of our true nature and potential. By accepting all parts of ourselves, we can experience a sense of freedom, and we can let go of external expectations that are not ours to fulfil. Our inner work can reveal to us how we have been living out of sync with our authenticity. And if we allow it, our wise internal power can guide us back to our truth.

The *panchamaya* koshas

Connecting with our wise power requires deep self-nurturing, integration and healing at all levels of our being so that we can be the most whole and truthful version of ourselves. Yoga teaches us that there are five layers of a human being called the *panchamaya koshas*: the physical body; the energy body; the mental body; the wisdom body; and the bliss body. The koshas move inwards from the dense, material, physical body to the subtle lightness at the core of our being. The layers are all interconnected and interdependent, and each layer is infused with universal divine intelligence. Also called life force or source energy, this is the same intelligence that allows the sun to rise, the flowers to bloom and the birds to sing. Some people call this intelligence mother nature, spirit, the divine, or God. Living our life in a way that sustains the vitality of all five koshas brings us back to wholeness.

The Physical Body *(annamaya kosha)*: This is the densest layer. It is the material, physical body that carries us through life. It is our skin, tissues, bones, cells and the complex web of interconnected bodily systems such as the cardiovascular, endocrine, musculoskeletal, immune, gastrointestinal and nervous systems. The physical body thrives on balance and equilibrium and is the gateway to discovering our inner landscape.

The Energy Body *(pranamaya kosha)*: This is the subtle energetic body. It relates to *prana*, the vital life force that gives our physical body life. It comes in through our breath and flows through the many inner channels and energy centres, circulating and distributing vitality to all aspects of our being, right down to our cells. With practice, we can become more aware of the subtle energy that makes up our being. Practices like breathwork (pranayama) and energy healing (such as reiki) can help us to remove energy blocks and create conditions that support our energy to flow freely, resourcing ourselves with vitality and vibrant power.

The Mental Body *(manomaya kosha)*: This nuanced layer relates to our mind, thoughts and emotions. The mind can be our best friend or our worst enemy. When we understand the qualities of the mind, we can develop practices to befriend our mind and find mental clarity, focus, creativity and inspiration that serve us in carrying out our purpose and living our lives with wisdom and meaning.

The Wisdom Body *(vijnanamaya kosha)*: This is our seat of wisdom, intuition, gut instinct or inner knowing. This layer of our being speaks to us in sensations, feelings and whispers. When we connect to our wisdom body, we are guided for our higher good. This is our inner power to help us navigate the challenges in life. Once we cultivate this part of us, we can tap into an infinite well of guidance and support. In our Western world, much of our focus is on the body and the mind, and we have lost our indigenous connection to this inner power.

The Bliss Body *(anandamaya kosha)*: This is our innermost essence, where we can access an infinite well of peace, love, joy, pleasure, kindness and compassion. It is here we find a mysterious sense of oneness with the universe and a sense of what we came here to do in this life. When we abide in this part of ourselves, we can infuse all our thoughts and actions with the qualities of the bliss body.

THE KOSHAS: The five bodies

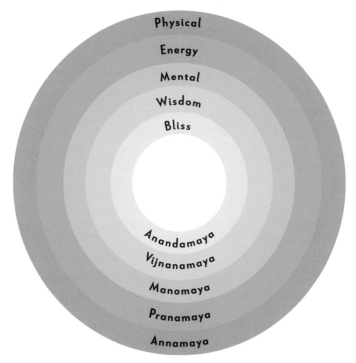

Physical

Energy

Mental

Wisdom

Bliss

Anandamaya

Vijnanamaya

Manomaya

Pranamaya

Annamaya

The path to purpose

Our journey to realising our true nature as wise
beings takes us through each layer, coming home to
our inner essence. As each layer is integrated, we feel
more supported to live with purpose. This path of self-
realisation is beautiful, but can be challenging as we get
to know ourselves fully and deeply. However, it is not
something to bring more fear, stress or burden into our
lives; it is a return to our sacredness, allowing us to let
go of some of our greatest fears and worries and fully

embrace our special gifts as we enter the second half of life. If you are ready, let us take this deep dive inwards through the layers of the koshas to meet our truest, wisest self.

Pearls of wisdom

- Ageing gives us the opportunity to learn, change, evolve and gain perspective, clarity and wisdom.
- We each have something wise and sacred to contribute to the world.
- Meaning and purpose come from love, connection and reaching our highest human potential, not from material possessions.
- We can work with our dosha to bring more balance into our lives.
- The expansiveness of vata offers us huge potential for emotional, spiritual and creative growth in midlife.
- Our individual and cultural attitude towards midlife might impact the severity of our hormonal symptoms in perimenopause and menopause.
- The biological changes in midlife facilitate our personal growth and transformation.
- Moving inwards through all the layers of our being, we meet our truest, wisest self.

CHAPTER THREE

The Wisdom of the Body

"*This is your body, your greatest gift,
pregnant with the wisdom you do not
hear, grief you thought was forgotten,
and the joy you have never known*"

MARION WOODMAN

Many of us have a complex relationship with our bodies. It took me until my mid-forties to realise that self-love is a choice we can consciously make. I remember a specific moment in my childhood, looking in a mirror and really liking my reflection. I was a sporty, strong and happy girl. But after a teenage heartbreak, my sense of self shifted. My teenage brain began to think that perhaps the boy would have loved me more if I had worn cooler clothes or better makeup, or if I fixed my hair better. I thought that I would be accepted and loved by others if I looked a certain way.

Critically, what I didn't realise was that without self-love and self-acceptance I was vulnerable, lacking boundaries and falling into relationships that were damaging to me. For too many years, I stayed in a relationship that was problematic. Feeling disempowered,

I tried to control what I could – my body – punishing it with a regime of overexercise and disordered eating. And through all of this turbulence, at not one moment did I pause and think that instead of looking for love outside I could choose to give love and acceptance to myself. It really could be that simple.

My slow journey towards healing began with yoga, a practice that brought me home to my body in the present moment, through embodiment, and helped me to cultivate a more loving relationship with my body. However, despite all this good work, as I began to witness my body shape shifting in my forties, I could sense my old controlling patterns creeping back in – the desire to obsess about food and exercise in order to cling to a more youthful version of my body.

It takes a lot of energy to be that hard on ourselves, and I didn't want to be that person again. I wanted to retain my energy for my passions, intuitive movement, hiking, creating art and painting. And then I had a light-bulb moment. What if I could simply consciously choose to stop criticising my body, flipping the negative thoughts in my head to begin to love my body as I would my best friend, showing it acceptance and gratitude for everything it does for me? Could I use the wise spiritual teachings I was offering others – of acceptance and love for their whole self – while I was going through my own perimenopausal transformation, and not regress back into my old patterns of dysfunction? I found that now more than ever, my practice of embodiment through yoga-inspired intuitive movement could support my nervous system and allow me to see the wonder in my body during this new phase of life. These are the teachings and practices I hope to share in order to encourage you to come home to your body.

The body is sacred

Our body is the vehicle through which we experience the world. All of our senses – sight, sound, touch, taste, smell, intuition – come through the body. It is a sacred vessel, holding all that we are, physically, energetically, mentally, emotionally and spiritually. And yet we spend so much of our lives rejecting our bodies through harsh self-criticism or by holding ourselves up against unrealistic and superficial ideas of physical beauty and perfection. As we watch our appearance shift and change in midlife, we have a *choice* either to finally embrace our bodies lovingly for all that they do for us or to engage in a mental war against our physicality and damage our connection to all the body can offer.

The body holds immense intelligence. By tuning into the language of the body, we can come to know the wisdom it holds. It speaks to us through felt sensations. And it is the gateway to our sense of well-being, offering us vital feedback all the time. If we battle our body through harsh self-criticism, or if we have become disassociated from our body as a result of trauma, we may miss out on all that we can feel and learn from our body.

The body does not lie

The mind and the body are interlinked through a stream of constant reciprocal communication. How we think and feel impacts the body, and our body influences how we think and feel. It is all interconnected, not separate, but at different times in our lives we might feel more in tune with the language of the mind than with the language of the body. The mind can communicate like a loud voice in our head, so it often takes more attention, while the language of the body is subtle until it needs to shout for us to take notice.

When we begin to listen to the language of the body, we can come into rhythm with ourselves at a much deeper level. Establishing a relationship with our body is a fundamental first step in getting to know ourselves better. It can teach us a lot about how we really feel about things and where we might be holding our burdens. Each part of our body is related to our psyche. Our emotions manifest as physical sensations, such as butterflies in our tummy, tension in our neck, a tight chest or a shallow breath. Whether we can recognise and respond to these signals from the body will depend on our sense of embodiment.

Having a clear awareness of our body allows us to feel anchored. From this grounded place, we can start to remember what it was that we came into the world to do. Being in right relationship with the body helps us to access and trust our gut instinct. How we feel about our bodies can inhibit our intuition, decision-making capabilities and boundary setting. Therefore, taking care of our bodies helps us to act from a place of clarity and balance so that we may become a more positive force for good in the world. Thích Nhất Hạnh, the Buddhist spiritual leader, taught that 'when you take care of yourself you are practically taking care of the world'.[1] Self-care begins with *embodiment*.

Being embodied

Embodiment is the degree to which we are fully in our bodies, receiving the felt sensations. When we are not fully present in our bodies, we are disconnected from the signals and messages the body wants us to hear. Living in our bodies without a sense of embodiment greatly impacts our ability to have self-awareness, to take care of ourselves and to maintain healthy boundaries. By contrast, noticing the felt senses in the body allows us to know how we feel and to establish what we need. This is how we develop awareness. For each of us, our sense of embodiment will determine the extent to which we can feel and receive the information from the body, process it, and then, if needed, take action. This is critical for our well-being, as it empowers us to take care of our own needs.

Modern life does not help embodiment

We ask many things of our body on a daily basis, but how often are we paying attention to the body, noticing the sensations, signals and feelings and then responding appropriately? This is a major dysfunction of modern life that is not serving us. The pace and pressure of how we live takes us out the present moment and out of our bodies into a mind that is rooted in worries for the future or the wounds of the past. Constant use of screens and technology draws our focus deeply into a virtual world, disconnecting us further. Our mind has taken over and we have disengaged from the body or become disembodied, meaning that even though we are living in a body, we are not really there. As we move through the world in this way, it can feel like we are on autopilot. The mind is in charge and the body is a secondary consideration.

Our lifestyle has exacerbated this duality, separating mind and body and giving the mental voice more power. The bodymind was never intended to be separate. It needs integration for our wholeness and will affect how we take care of our physical needs, what movement we do, and how we nourish the body with our food choices.

An embodiment crisis at midlife

At midlife in particular, women are under a multitude of pressures and responsibilities. It is a complex time, when we might be sandwiched between our career, caring for children and caring for ageing parents or other relatives whilst also fulfilling our role as a partner, sister, friend and colleague. Juggling numerous roles with precious little time to tune into ourselves can cause us to further disconnect and ignore the language of our body. We can become vulnerable to unhealthy boundaries, allowing ourselves to neglect our own needs in favour of the needs of others. If we override the signals of our body to put the needs of others ahead of ourselves, this can lead over time to chronic physical pain and mental health issues. Lacking time to take care of ourselves, we might start to think that the body is letting us down. Instead of practising kindness and compassion towards the challenges facing our physicality during midlife, we can become resentful and full of self-loathing.

Embodiment helps us access our inner compass

A difficult relationship with our body will influence our connection with the deepest core of who we are. We each have an internal compass – that deep seat of knowing or the voice of intuitive wisdom that serves to guide us and keep us on the right path. It keeps us in flow with the right rhythm of our life. When we attune to it, we can find what gives us meaning and purpose in our lives. It is an inner superpower.

However, to hear the voice of intuition, we must be grounded in the present moment in our bodies. Otherwise, we are off imagining the future or the past versions of our life, and we will miss the signals of the inner voice. Becoming embodied involves taking baby steps to meet your body in the present moment, gently coming back to sensing and feeling the body again. Can we give ourselves a chance to befriend the vessel that carries us through life? To do this, we need to be able to go inwards and build up our 'interoception' – the sense of knowing how we feel (self-awareness) and being able to notice the sensations in our body and interpret what they mean. Embodiment and interoception support us in accessing our inner wisdom.

PRACTICE: The body scan

This is a practice we can do to explore our sense of embodiment. There is no right or wrong way to feel in this practice. If it is hard for you to notice the sensations in your body, please be kind to yourself. It can take time to reconnect with the body. Many people who have experienced pain and trauma can find it hard to be in their body. It may not feel safe. So please be gentle with yourself. If it doesn't feel safe for you to connect with your body right now, give yourself permission to skip the practice for the time being.

If you do feel ready, please find a comfortable seat with your feet on the ground. If the chair is high, place your feet on a cushion so they have something to rest on. You are welcome to take your shoes and socks off if you like or keep them on if you prefer. Closing the eyes can help us to move the focus inwards, but some people prefer to keep them open. It's your choice. If it feels safe to close your eyes, go ahead. Now, take a moment to notice your body. Can you sense the touch of the clothes on your skin? Notice the parts of your body that are touching the chair. Notice where the body is connected to the support beneath you. Can you notice the feet on the ground or the cushion?

Do you notice any sensation in the toes or the feet? Can you feel the soles of the feet resting? Can you notice the heels? All of the toes? The ankles? Allow the awareness to move up the legs, noticing any sensations in the legs. Where do you feel it? Maybe the lower legs or the thighs? Can you begin to notice the buttocks resting on the chair? Is there any sensation here?

Can you notice any sensation in the front of the hips? Or the back of the hips? Noticing the natural curves of the spine, can you sense the arch of the lower back, the middle spine and upper back and the curve at the back of the neck? As you notice the back body, just observe any sensations that arise — any tension or tight spots you can feel. Is there any part of the back that feels tense? Then allow the awareness to move to the belly. Notice any sensations around the abdomen. Can you begin to soften the whole belly? Maybe you can feel gentle movement in the belly as you breathe or maybe you feel the breath further up in the ribs or the chest. Just notice what you notice.

Can you move the awareness to the shoulders, noticing how they feel? Notice the back of the neck and the throat, what you feel in this area, if anything. Now moving the awareness to your face, can you notice your chin? Your lips? Your right cheek? Left cheek? Allow the awareness to move to the head. Can you sense the hair on your head? Just observe any sensations that you feel. Then when you are ready, start to feel your arms and your legs again and bring some gentle movement into the toes and the fingers. Take a moment to notice how you feel, without judgement. You can return to this practice any time you want to come back to your body.

The systems of the body

The body is our home, and it is crucial that it is somewhere we feel comfortable. If we can belong in our body, this will help us have a sense of belonging in other places. The bodymind is an intricate system that thrives on homeostasis or equilibrium. Much like nature, the bodymind is a beautiful garden of parts that are connected to form an amazing ecosystem. Each system of the body (such as the cardiovascular, endocrine, musculoskeletal, immune, gastrointestinal and nervous systems) has its own function to maintain the harmony of the entire ecosystem. Imbalances in one system can cause a lack of equilibrium in another, and over time may manifest as an accumulation of *dis-ease* or disharmony in the form of physical illness. Our well-being is reliant on a unified bodymind to oversee the functioning of all of our parts. The mind and the body communicate together through our nervous system. This is like our own electrical wiring that sends and receives information all over the body. The nervous system is constantly monitoring our sense of safety and well-being so that we can adapt to survive. By exploring the nervous system, we gain some insight into how the mind and our body are programmed to interact, react and take action.

Our nervous system

The central nervous system (CNS) is located in the brain and the spine. It functions like the central processing unit in a computer. It processes information and decides what actions to take. The CNS takes in information from the peripheral nervous system (PNS), which is located in all of the nerves that branch out of the brain and the spinal cord and reach all over the body. Like an interconnected web, the CNS creates the lines of communication between the brain, the spine and the whole of the body. It is the controller, so when it has processed information and made a decision, it then communicates the action needed to the whole of the body through the PNS.

The PNS is like a courier, delivering the message of action all over the body to the cells, joints, muscles and deep connective tissue. This process of communication happens so rapidly that we are not really aware of it until it impacts our behaviour and responses. Contained within the peripheral nervous system we have the autonomic nervous system (ANS), which is subdivided into three parts that we may be more familiar with: the enteric nervous system; the sympathetic nervous system; and the parasympathetic nervous system.

Our gut health – the enteric nervous system

The enteric nervous system is the largest part of the peripheral nervous system, and it is the connection between the gut and the brain. Our gut is our largest sensory organ, with over 100 million neurons that tune into our inner landscape and communicate with the brain through nerve fibres. The vagus nerve is the fastest and most important route from the gut to the brain.[2] The gut lets the brain know if we feel safe or if we feel threatened or fearful.

The 'microbiome', which is all the bacteria in the gut, is fundamental to ensuring these messages can be received and interpreted. Therefore, a healthy microbiome helps the function of our enteric nervous system. The food we use to fuel our body impacts our gut health and in turn our nervous system. When our microbiome is disturbed, the connection to the brain is disturbed. So the gut plays a vital role in our well-being and is often called our 'second brain'. Serotonin is the neurotransmitter responsible for memory, regulating mood, digestion and sleep – all of which can be affected in midlife, and 90 per cent of our serotonin is produced in the gut. Therefore, by looking after our gut – choosing food that supports our gut health – we encourage the healthy production of serotonin that is critical to supporting our health at this time in our life. Foods that tend to support gut health include plant-based foods, foods that are high in fibre (including fruit, vegetables, nuts, wholegrains and pulses), live yoghurt and fermented foods. Processed foods tend not to support gut health.

Scientist Guilia Enders says that stress is the most important stimulus for our gut, potentially 'changing the weather in the gut' – the microbiome. Enders' work shows that the health of the gut suffers when we experience long-term stress, because stress of any kind inhibits digestion.[3] Whenever the gut senses stress, it communicates this to the brain and the CNS, activating the sympathetic nervous system, more commonly known as 'fight or flight'.

The stress response

When the CNS receives the signal that we don't feel safe, stress hormones like adrenaline and cortisol are released to activate the sympathetic nervous system and help us use stored energy to either stay and fight off the perceived threat or run away and escape from danger. The stress response immediately suppresses the systems of the body that are not vital to our survival in this present moment – like digestion, reproduction and our immune system – by reducing their blood supply. Instead, our heart rate and blood pressure increase to pump extra blood to the bigger muscles of the body in order to help us fight or run away.

Everything else that is happening now in the body is to help us survive the threat. So our breathing becomes faster and shallower to get more oxygen quickly in order to help us fight or flee; our pupils dilate and our perspective becomes narrower and more focused; our body temperature rises and we sweat more to keep cool; we can either lose control of our bladder or bowels or become constipated, holding things in until we feel it is safer to release; our senses are heightened to keep us on high alert; our long-term memory function is affected, as it is no longer critical to our immediate survival; our decision-making is less rational and more short term; and our mouth feels dry, as salvia production is stopped because digestion has been inhibited. All of these changes serve to help us stay alive. It is only when we perceive ourselves to be out of danger that we can return to feeling a sense of safety that allows the stress response to be deactivated.

The relaxation response

Relaxation is necessary to switch off the stress response. Herbert Benson coined the term 'the relaxation response' to describe the critical function of the para-sympathetic nervous system (PNS).[4] This is the body-mind response designed to help us rest and digest and come back into balance after enduring stress. After fighting or fleeing, the body needs time to recover and build up its energy reserves, allowing all the systems of the body to move back into balance. In this relaxed state, our heart rate slows down and our blood pressure drops. Our breathing becomes slower and deeper. The muscles begin to relax. Our digestive system starts to resume, producing saliva again to help with this. The blood supply returns to the reproductive organs, encouraging fertility. And it is only in this relaxed state that we can experience deep restoration and sleep that promote healthy immunity and facilitate the growth of our cells. Note that critically *a felt sense of safety* must be experienced to allow the body to move into the relaxation response.

The role of the vagus nerve

Remember the vagus nerve, the important communicator between the gut and the brain – this is what stimulates the relaxation response. Called 'vagal toning', it encourages the felt sense of safety in the body. The vagus nerve runs from the brain to the abdomen through the heart and the diaphragm – our primary breathing muscle. Practices like deep belly breathing, laughing, singing or chanting will very quickly help us to feel more relaxed – as they involve using the diaphragm to tone the vagus nerve. Now, as we have seen, relaxation is crucial for enabling the body to recover and come back to balance after stress. But furthermore, when we are relaxed, we can feel safe enough to experience embodiment and interoception – noticing our felt sensations, feelings and emotions from a grounded, safe state.

The freeze response

Apart from relaxation, the parasympathetic nervous system plays another vital role in our survival. When our brain thinks the body will not survive a threat by fighting or fleeing, another option is available to protect us. This is the 'freeze response', and it is one way the body can respond to trauma. Stephen Porges, an American neuroscientist, developed polyvagal theory, which proposes that the vagus nerve has two branches.[5]

Put simply, the first branch is the dorsal vagal root, which shuts down the body in the freeze response, causing us to become immobile or to disassociate. The second branch is the ventral vagus root, which can have a more calming influence on the nervous system. Dorsal vagal shutdown provides an important protection mechanism that can be experienced on a spectrum from mild disassociation from the body to becoming completely frozen. At the extreme end of this spectrum, the body shuts down, we are unable to move or speak, and endorphins are released to manage pain and prepare us for death. However, milder reactions can see us become somewhat disembodied and disassociated from the sensations in our body. When this happens, we may not be able to know how we feel, we may have trouble connecting and feeling the sensations within us, and we may feel unable to take the right actions to meet our needs.

Many of us who have experienced trauma, no matter how old the trauma, can still be living with a degree of disassociation. For some of us, the response to trauma will be more severe and can lead to post-traumatic stress disorder (PTSD). This can be very distressing, as the memory of the trauma is often relived through flashbacks and nightmares, retriggering the nervous system response, time and time again. We can heal from trauma and can come back into healthy relationship with our bodies, but it may take time, patience and working safely with a specialised trauma therapist.

The impact of chronic long-term stress

Not all stress is bad, and sometimes we need a little pressure to get tasks done. But each of these protective responses – fight, flight or freeze – is only intended to be activated for a short period of time, until the threat subsides, we feel safe again, and the body can start to return to balance through the activation of the relaxation response.

The bodily systems can endure the symptoms of these protective modes for a short period of time without long-term consequences. But what if the protective mode is chronic and there is no release of the symptoms? Over time, this leads to imbalances that culminate in disease. Chronic stress and trauma are major inhibitors of wellness at all layers of our being and are now correlated with many Western lifestyle diseases, including heart disease, stroke, high blood pressure, adrenal fatigue and burnout. And past stressors, emotional pain or trauma may still be held in the body, influencing us in the present.

Bessel van der Kolk, in his groundbreaking book *The Body Keeps the Score*, shows that the body can hold on to past stress and trauma long after the events have passed, and that this has long-term consequences for our well-being.[6] Furthermore, the research of Canadian-American paediatrician Nadine Burke Harris links our adverse childhood experiences (ACE) – which can include psychological, physical, and sexual abuse as well as exposure to substance abuse, mental illness, violence, and parental incarceration in childhood – to toxic stress that has negative effects on our health as adults.[7] Therefore, we can be carrying the impact of our negative early life experiences into midlife if we don't allow ourselves time and space to heal and let go.

It is never too late to heal

The resilience of our nervous system, sometimes called the 'window of tolerance', relates to how easily we can switch between the stress response and the relaxation response. How well we bounce back from stressful life events depends on our unique individual experiences, early intervention, our support systems and the quality of our social relationships. When we understand and recognise why we think and act as we do, we empower ourselves with the wisdom of self-awareness that goes a long way to helping us to heal. It is possible to heal the impact of trauma, and it is never too late. We can work slowly, gently and safely in a trauma-informed way to start to build this connection to our bodies again. Working to enhance our sense of embodiment is a great first step towards empowering ourselves to heal.

CASE STUDY: Emma, a stay-at-home mother of four children, was in her mid-forties when her husband, Darren, suddenly asked for a divorce. He told her he had met a woman named Gloria at work. They had been having an affair for about a year and now Darren was going to move in with her. The news came as a massive shock to Emma. When she came to me for yoga therapy, she was deeply upset and very stressed. She had no appetite and had lost a lot of weight. Emma did not want her marriage to end, and she was finding it hard to accept what was happening. Her sleep was disturbed, and she was mentally and physically exhausted. She was unable to relax, her mind was anxious, and she was experiencing panic attacks. With her body under so much physical and emotional stress, her immune system was compromised and she was getting lots of chest infections. Her doctor had prescribed her both sleeping tablets and antidepressants. During our yoga sessions, she was very hard on herself. She didn't feel she was coping well, and she was worried about the effect on her children. Her nervous system was overwhelmed by the shock of the divorce, and she had become disassociated from her body. It was difficult for her to feel and notice the felt sensations in her body, and she felt relaxation was impossible. We began to work gently, moving together while we talked, careful to avoid long silences that would allow her thoughts to take over. We worked gently with her breathing to help with her panic attacks. Even though she was experiencing deep pain and sadness, Emma had a great sense of humour and she laughed and cried during our sessions. Yoga became a safe space for her to release whatever she needed to release. Very gradually, she started to feel safer in her body. Becoming more embodied, she started to notice the sensations in her body more and she became better able to take care of herself, making sure she ate and trying to get more rest. Slowly, her nervous system began to settle and she could enjoy relaxation at the end of yoga. Sometimes she even fell asleep. Her body was craving this deep rest to facilitate restoration, recovery and healing. As she started to feel safer in her body, her mind became less anxious and her nervous system started to regulate. Her mood improved, and gradually she found a sense of acceptance with the end of her marriage. Over time, her enthusiasm for life returned and she became excited to make future plans.

Our beliefs change the body's chemistry

Neuroscience shows us that the body responds in the exact same way to a perceived threat as it does to a 'real' threat. The threat can be coming from a thought or from a fear of a future event or something that may never even happen. But the body will respond to the fearful thought by activating the stress response. The beliefs that we tell ourselves change the chemistry in the body. The body responds in two main ways to the beliefs of the mind – with either the stress response or the relaxation response. If the mind signals to the brain that we are in danger, the stress response is activated through the sympathetic nervous system. If the mind signals to the brain that we are safe, the relaxation response kicks in through the parasympathetic nervous system.

The power of thoughts

Our mind has the power to make our biochemistry go out of balance. American developmental biologist Bruce Lipton calls this the 'biology of belief'.[8] We have a spectrum of thoughts, emotions and feelings that move us like a pendulum towards fear or towards love. We will explore the power of our thoughts in greater detail in Chapter 6. For now, we can simply begin to realise that our thoughts – by moving us more towards love or fear – greatly influence our nervous system and the biochemical reaction in the body. As we lean into fear, the body activates the stress response to help us survive, and as we lean into love, the relaxation response is switched on as the body feels safe and free from threat.

How we live our daily lives can cause us chronic, low-grade stress, putting us in a sympathetic activation that will be reflected in the chemistry of the body. The root cause of our stress is irrelevant; chemically, we will respond in the same way once the stress response is activated, releasing the stress hormones. This means that even if our fears are not true or real, once we perceive something as unsafe, fear manifests as thoughts and feelings, and we signal to the brain that we are not safe. Likewise, if the fear is held in the body from past trauma, the body communicates the perceived current lack of safety to the brain and the stress response is activated.

The nervous system is designed to alternate back and forth with relative ease. It is a resilient system, and we can endure short-term stressors and then recover through rest and relaxation, with the chemistry of the body coming back into balance or equilibrium. But we are not designed for chronic stress. This is damaging for our whole being over time, as the chemistry of the body is thrown out of balance for too long, and without enough opportunities for restoration and recovery.

The normalisation of stress

Most of us do not even realise we are experiencing the stress response. We think of stress as some colossal, monumental life event. When asked if we are stressed, we might say no. But if we are asked if we feel under pressure in our lives, our answer might be quite different. Over time, being under pressure is stressful, and it activates the same chemical reaction in the body that stress does, regardless of which description or language we accept. The body responds the same way.

The same can be said of trauma, and most of us will have experienced some trauma in our lives. In fact, we have all experienced a collective trauma: the Covid-19 pandemic. The word 'trauma' will be interpreted differently by each of us. Whether or not we acknowledge that we have been through something traumatic, if we have, then the chemistry in the body will have been altered. We may not realise we are stressed until we try to relax. If we have been living with chronic stress for some time, then it becomes our default mode. It becomes normalised for us to feel that way, because it has been so long since we have felt any differently, and it may be frightening and challenging to experience deep, profound relaxation.

PRACTICE: Restorative supported supta baddha konasana

Restorative yoga is a wonderful practice to reset the nervous system. Using lots of props like cushions and blankets, we can fully support the body in passive stretches to completely let go and offer the nervous system a chance for deep rest and restoration. If you find it difficult to relax, you may want to move your body a little bit before you come to rest in this restorative yoga pose. This pose is called *supported supta baddha konasana or reclined bound angle pose.* It can be useful to do before bed to help prepare the body for sleep, or you can use it during the day whenever you feel like you need to take a few minutes to rest and recharge.

Start by creating a raised base using some yoga blocks or books, and then rest a bolster or stack of pillows or cushions on a horizontal slant. Make sure they are steady and will hold the weight of your back. Place one or two folded blankets at the top of your bolster that you will use to support your head. Roll another blanket up that you will use as a support for under your knees.

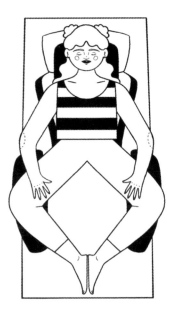

· Sit with your back facing the supported bolster and move in close so that your tailbone is right at the start of the bolster. Don't sit on the bolster. Slowly recline yourself onto the support. Make sure your head is fully supported with enough blankets that your chin can be slightly tucked into your chest to keep your neck long. Support all of your joints. For your comfort and safety, don't allow them to hang in mid-air. You can place a cushion under each elbow and wrist. Place the rolled-up blanket under your knees and a soft blanket under your feet. Cover your whole body in a blanket to keep yourself warm and cosy. It can feel very soothing to gently tuck either side of the blanket under your head to create a little nest for your head. Comfort is crucial to relaxation. Make any little adjustments that you need in order to feel fully supported. You can place an eye pillow or a light scarf over your eyes. Allow your whole body to melt into the support beneath you and feel yourself being held. Find a comfortable breath and take a few minutes to deeply relax.

Pearls of wisdom

- ○ Our body is sacred and intelligent and holds great wisdom.
- ○ How we feel about our bodies can inhibit our intuition, decision-making capabilities and boundary setting.
- ○ Becoming embodied, and developing an awareness of the sensations in the body, allows us to connect with who we are and recognise the signals when things are out of balance.
- ○ Past stressors, emotional pain or trauma may still be held in the body.
- ○ Midlife is a time for healing old wounds.
- ○ Cultivating safety in the body and mind is essential for relaxation and healing.

CHAPTER FOUR

Moving Wisely

"*Movement is the song of the body*"
VANDA SCARAVELLI

n my late twenties, I finally found the courage to leave a damaging relationship. However, this experience had a huge impact on my self-worth and my sense of self. I was disconnected from my body and my boundaries were unhealthy. I didn't trust myself, ignoring my instincts and intuition time and time again. Without doing the inner work that I needed to heal myself, I made choices in my life that were out of alignment with who I was, and I walked straight into another relationship that was toxic. I developed irritable bowel syndrome as my body screamed to get my attention. Ignoring my inner voice, I tried to numb myself with alcohol.

When I took my first yoga class, I felt like my life was a mess. Slowly, however, this practice of conscious movement brought me back in touch with myself. As I practised yoga, I became more embodied and more myself, and I started to become aware of my patterns of self-sabotage. Yoga helped me to continue to heal and to connect back with my authentic self. By helping me to safely release stress and tension and to regulate my nervous system and my emotions, it led to a profound shift in my well-being at all levels – physical, mental, emotional and spiritual. Most importantly, consciously moving with the breath helped me to learn to trust myself and find my inner power. After I experienced first-hand how yoga could be therapeutic, I knew that my purpose was to share this practice with others.

Coming home to ourselves

Mindful movement can help us to come home to our bodies and to meet ourselves in the present moment. When we move, we can notice how it feels to be in our bodies, we can feel playful and curious, and we can create more comfort and pleasure in the body. With the shifts in midlife, wise movement is a gift to our body, mind and spirit. By moving with intention, we can give ourselves what we need – safety, comfort, vitality, energy and inspiration. Using movement, we can tailor our practice to meet our changing physical needs and cultivate more self-kindness, self-compassion and self-love as we transition to midlife.

Movement as medicine

If we are holding on to tension, worry, stress and the imprint of trauma, it will be impossible to relax.

Movement can offer us a way to let go. We can learn a lot from animals about releasing tension. Every day, on my regular walk with my springer spaniel, Bella, we pass a gated house with two huge Bernese mountain dogs who bark loudly when we pass, protecting their territory. As we approach this house, my dog prepares for this stressful encounter by activating her sympathetic nervous system, getting ready to go into battle and to defend herself from attack. She goes into fight mode, barking back at the dogs.

But after the few short seconds it takes to walk by, she has a big shake, letting go of the encounter, and gets back to sniffing the grass. The 'shake off' is a key step in helping her deal with the stress, allowing her nervous system to release the build-up of tension and to come back into a balanced state in a matter of seconds. She intuitively uses the movement to release and let go. We can learn from animals and use movement as a safe release to let go of the imprint of the physical or emotional stress in the body and to help us to come back into balance.

We cannot relax under duress. A sense of safety must be cultivated first. The first place we need to feel this safety is in the home of our body. The mind needs to feel safe in the body, and the body needs the mind to feel this safety to allow the nervous system to activate relaxation. Movement offers us a pathway to create a safe release and let go of what the body is holding.

Many psychotherapists have recognised that traditional talk therapies that ask clients to revisit difficult situations can be retraumatising, triggering the stress response once again. A combined approach using somatic movement can help to offer a way to release and heal old wounds through the body in a way that talk therapy alone may not. Used in this way, movement becomes therapeutic and medicinal. We may have experienced this at times when we took a walk or hike with a friend and talked about what was bothering us. We can feel lighter afterwards, as the motion moves the emotional issues out of our physical tissues.

A regular movement practice is a powerful tool for healing and offers profound freedom and space in the body. Movement can offer us a way to release the build-up of tension, pressure and stress to create more space, comfort and relaxation in the body. This tones down the stress response, bringing the nervous system back to balance. Releasing through movement, we allow the energy within us to flow more freely and reach the places in the body where it needs to go, increasing vitality. When we hold on to stress in the body, our energy becomes blocked and stuck, and this accumulates in the form of more tension, which can lead to chronic pain and illness. When we move wisely, with the intention of releasing what the body is holding, we can begin to move towards freedom and peace.

PRACTICE: Shaking it off

This is a very simple movement practice you can do at any time of the day to feel looser and lighter in your body and help to shake off tension and stress. Stand with your feet hip-width apart. Softly bend the elbows and begin to shake both hands about 5 to 10 times. Now, relaxing the arms by your side, shake both arms up and down about 5 to 10 times. Bring the hands to your hips, lift one leg, begin to shake or kick the leg loose and then swap legs, alternating legs about 5 to 10 times. You can hold on to a wall or a chair for balance. Then gently sway the body from side to side about 5 to 10 times — you can let the arms move freely as you move When you are finished, take a moment to roll your shoulders up and back and move your head from side to side. Allow the body to find stillness. Notice how you feel now.

How wise movement tones the nervous system

Recall the location of the central nervous system (CNS) – in the brain and spine. The spinal cord, contained in the spine, houses the nerves that send and receive messages between the brain and the body. The peripheral nervous system (PNS) branches out from the CNS, travelling everywhere else in the body. If we can create length and space in our spine, this will tone the nervous system, and creating comfort and ease in the whole of the body will enhance the integration of the whole nervous system.

The yoga tradition says that life-force energy flows through 72,000 channels or pathways in the body called *nadis*. Traditional Chinese Medicine (TCM) describes similar energy pathways, called 'meridians', that support the uninterrupted flow of vital energy known in TCM as *chi* or *qi*. The ancient yogis said that the most important channel is the *sushumna nadi*, which runs down the centre of the body through the spine. They believed that if our energy pathways are blocked, we may develop difficulties in our physical and mental health. We will take a deeper dive into the subtle energy system of the body in the next chapter, but for now, just consider that we are made of energy and that we need to move our bodies to allow energy to flow to where it needs to go. By releasing the imprint of stress, tension and tightness, we feel more comfort and vitality in our body, because we are facilitating the life-force energy to flow without constriction. Developing the health of the spine by moving in different directions supports the optimum function of the energy channels and our nervous system.

Movement creates space for the breath

The life-force energy that the body needs enters through our breath. Movement is then the process which circulates this energy to the organs, tissues and spaces inside us that need vitality. The breath enters our lungs, and if our posture is contracted, we restrict how much air we can take in. We need space and length in our body to help our lungs to function. Through movement, we can create more space in the body for the breath to reach the deeper parts of the lungs.

The importance of being comfortable in the body

Pain or the experience of discomfort in the body, through injury or illness, affects our mood, well-being and relationships with others. We need to gently move our bodies every day and regularly throughout the day. This is especially important as we move into midlife, to support the health of the joints and keep a sense of juiciness in the body. One of the most common complaints I hear from women moving towards midlife is that everything in the body feels stiffer. Remember that vata dosha is making the body become drier as we age. This is part of the natural ageing process. Moving little and often, especially as we get older, is great for keeping a sense of liquidness flowing in the body.

Our lifestyle can help or hinder how stiff the body feels. Sitting for long periods, including when driving, contracts and compresses the body. We thrive on giving the body length, space and expansion. Our sedentary lives rarely provide enough movement for our body to feel a sense of openness. So, to feel as good as we possibly can, we must incorporate plenty of opportunities to move and liberate our bodies. We should not wait for movement to be prescribed by a doctor. It is good to use movement wisely, as preventative medicine, to keep us juicy for as long as possible. However, overexercise is also a form of self-harm. It can damage our bodies and deplete our energy. We need to have the right amount of movement and the right type of movement to meet our individual needs. Wise movement should help us to get to know ourselves better, help us to feel comfort and space in our body, and sustain our energy rather than drain it.

CASE STUDY: Belinda was in her late forties, with a lot on her plate. She was a single mother, an educator and studying for her master's. Both her parents were elderly, with long-term health problems. She lived close to them and spent a lot of her time bringing them to their individual health check-ups. Belinda was diagnosed with fibromyalgia, a condition that causes chronic pain and fatigue. She came to my general group yoga class. The class was very dynamic, with a focus on building strength and flexibility. Belinda told me she loved the class and felt it helped her to feel less pain, but that afterwards she felt so tired she would spend a day in bed to recover. She was going to two or three other yoga classes a week, pushing herself in very challenging poses even if they felt hard, and afterwards she was very fatigued and needed more rest to recover. I was concerned that her yoga practice was draining her energy rather than sustaining or giving her more energy. I invited her to come to me for a few complementary yoga therapy sessions to see if we could adapt the tools of yoga more wisely for her to help her manage pain without causing more fatigue. Over the course of five sessions, we adopted the approach of 'less is more'. We found what poses felt good for her body and offered her more relief from pain. We introduced more relaxation tools to nourish her energy, and we explored how she could include more kindness and self-compassion so she did not overdo it. Belinda said she could feel the difference and was more confident of how she could adapt her practice at home and in the group class to do what was right for her own body. By taking a more individual approach, she could use yoga to give her more nourishment rather than depleting her energy.

Movement regulates our emotions

Physical movement can help the emotional landscape to shift and change. As we move, we release pent-up emotions. Movement increases endorphins, the feel-good hormones. Even though it is sometimes hard to get motivated to move, we always feel better afterwards. Becoming conscious about our lifestyle, we can make small changes that result in big differences. Consider how we can limit our time sitting or driving for long periods and instead take time to move freely. During midlife, as parents or carers, we may be in and out of the car constantly during the day. Ironically, a lot of this might be driving the kids to their structured movement activities like sports and dance classes. While the children get a chance to move and feel good, we are often stuck sitting waiting and getting stiffer. This lack of movement leads to an accumulation of pressure that can manifest emotionally as frustration, restlessness, anger and resentment. If we have enough time to move and create the freedom and space the body craves, we start to feel more content, with more emotional regulation.

Using movement to bring balance to the body

Having a balanced nervous system provides the optimum condition in which we can heal our body and create positive change in our lives. Coming back into balance should be the intention of our movement for modern life. If we are already out of balance, we can unconsciously choose practices that exacerbate our imbalances. This is the principal of the law of attraction in physics – that like attracts like. So often we are attracted to exercise practices that can give us more of what we have already. Let's revisit the three doshas again. Our health and well-being are optimised when we live in a way that brings our predisposed predominant dosha into balance and harmony.[1] When we understand our individual tendency for imbalance, we can choose to tailor our movement in a way that wisely brings us back into harmony. If you completed the dosha questionnaire in Chapter 2, you may now have an idea of your dosha. Movement practices that offset our dosha can bring us into wholeness. Here are some examples in the context of yoga styles.

Movement to balance excess vata: If we have an excess of vata, we have a lot of air and ether in our system. This can be expansive and very creative, but can also make us feel like we are in our heads a lot and less embodied.

We can be overthinkers and tend to ruminate. This can stop us from seeing things through to the end and completing tasks. Vata people have so many ideas, but find it hard to ground them into action. Remembering that the qualities of vata are light and dry, it can be really useful to increase the elements of kapha (earth and water) to ground and offset vata. It may be difficult to get vata to drop down to kapha straight away. We need to meet ourselves where we are at and work our way down to the floor. If we like a lot of standing movement, start here and do some dynamic movement, moving into pitta to be able to begin to get to kapha practices that are slower, less heating and more grounding. For example, yoga poses that are seated or lying on the floor will give us a sense of being rooted and grounded. This can take us out of our heads and move us into our physical body, allowing us to feel more centred, calm and steady. As midlife is the vata stage of life, using more cooling, grounded movement will help to release pitta and balance excess vata.

Movement for excess pitta: With this dosha, we already have a lot of fire and heat in the body. We may be very orientated towards results and goals, and attracted to physically demanding, sweaty exercise that diminishes our energy levels and puts more heat into the body instead of restoring, healing and replenishing our vessel. To balance pitta, we might benefit from more cooling, slower, gentler movement practices. We might need to burn off some excess heat before we can come to slower practices, however. If you have a lot of pitta, start with some dynamic movement to give yourself what you like, but then start to incorporate movement on all fours, seated and lying down. Gentle, fluid, watery movements will have a cooling effect to invite more kapha into the body to balance pitta.

Movement for excess kapha: If we have too much earth and water, we might be lethargic, feeling stuck and not moving enough. Introducing a little more heat with pitta practices will ignite the fire of transformation and move us into action. But we might need to start slowly and gently to meet our kapha before building up to a more dynamic standing practice that can balance kapha.

The approach of yoga therapy

By considering the doshas in our movement practices, we can give our body exactly what it needs. In yoga therapy, we use intelligent sequencing to match the practices with the client. Every pose must be a good fit for the person and their needs in the present moment. The movement must fit the person and not the other way around. In tailoring a session, a yoga therapist will consider what poses will help achieve the desired results for the client. Do they need to slow down, or would dynamic movement be more appropriate to take them out of their head and move them more into their body? We tailor the practice to give the body more of what it is lacking and not more of what is already overloaded in the system. The amazing thing is that every one of us can learn to become more in tune with what we need and offer this to ourselves.

When we start to listen to the language of our body, we come into rhythm. This might involve *undoing* rather than doing. As we become wiser with our use of movement, we don't cause any strain or pain. Here we experience less disturbances in our body and mind, which frees up more space to connect with our intuition and our soul. By calming the elements that are out of balance, we can start nourishing and repairing the body, helping it to feel better, not worse, by moving wisely and aligning with our rhythm.

Getting moving

If a regular movement practice has not been part of your life for a long time, you may at first find that moving and stretching feels hard, tight and uncomfortable. You may notice a lack of comfort in the body. The muscles may not be flexible or strong. You may feel sore and fatigued, and it may feel easier to just sit back down again. However, if you continue to move gently and often, the body starts to loosen up surprisingly quickly. And as more space is created in the body, the movement becomes enjoyable and less like a chore or punishment. It becomes something you crave and *want* to do rather than something you *must* do. When we are new to moving and unsure of how to get started, structured classes with a guide or a teacher can be a helpful starting point. Mindful movement like dance, yoga and tai chi can offer a structure for you to begin to relate to your body in the present moment, encourage interoception, and get to know yourself better.

PRACTICE: Moving to become more embodied

This is a gentle movement sequence to help you ground your awareness in your physical body and become more embodied. This practice can be done on all fours or standing – if you have knee or wrist pain you might prefer to practise standing.

If coming onto all fours, put a blanket under your knees for comfort. To begin, place your wrists under your shoulders and your knees under your hips, about hip-width apart. To prevent the weight dumping into your wrists, spread your fingers with your middle finger pointing forward and press the back of the knuckles into the earth. Allow a micro-bend in your elbows and roll your upper arms in slightly. Gaze downwards, keeping your neck in line with your spine. This pose is called *table* and the spine is neutral (figure 1 on p104).

When you inhale, bring your bottom slightly back towards your heels and allow your heart to lift and your gaze to move upwards, perhaps noticing the arch in your mid-back. Be careful not to overarch the neck, as this compresses the vertebrae; just move your head in a range of motion that feels comfortable for you. This position is called *cow* pose (figure 2 on p104).

As you exhale, press your hands into the earth and hug your navel into your spine as you round your back, letting your head relax in between your arms. Only move the head in a range of motion that feels good for your neck. This position is called *cat* pose (figure 3 on p104).

If you feel comfortable in each part of these movements, begin to link them with your breath and move in and out of cat–cow about 5–10 times. You are welcome to close your eyes and move your awareness inwards, noticing how the movement feels inside your body. What felt sensations do you notice? How does the movement feel for your spine? Where do you feel any tension or tightness? Where do you feel like you need more space in your body?

After you have moved through cat–cow a few times, bring your awareness to your tailbone. Begin to draw circles with your tailbone, allowing your hips to circle (figure 4 on p104). Start with small gentle movements and then gradually allow the circles to become bigger. Notice how this movement feels for your body. What sensations do you notice? How do your hips feel?

If you are comfortable, you might like to bring some fluid circular movements into your upper back, shoulders, neck and head, moving your body in a way that feels good for you. Continue to connect with your breath. Tune inwards and allow your body to guide you intuitively. When you are ready, you might like to explore moving the hips in the other direction. After a couple of minutes, allow the movement to slow down and notice how you feel now.

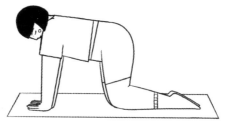

fig 1.

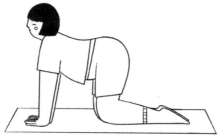

fig 2

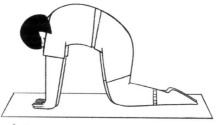

fig 3

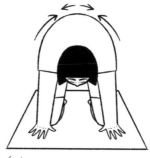

fig 4.

Connecting to our core

The core is our seat of inner power, strength and action, and is located below the ribcage. It is made up of a group of muscles including the pelvic floor muscles, abdominal muscles, back muscles and diaphragm – our primary breathing muscle. After pregnancy, many of us can lose connection with our core, as the muscles feel weaker, particularly in the pelvic floor. Some of us find it more difficult to regain that connection post-partum. As we move into midlife, establishing our reconnection to our core is very important if we are to protect our balance and stability, prevent back injury, prolapse and incontinence, and enjoy sex. A healthy connection here also feels empowering, as we feel strong and ready for action. It is worth seeing a women's health physiotherapist or a yoga or Pilates therapist to get a tailored programme to build up your core and pelvic floor.

PRACTICE: Gentle pelvic tilts and thrust

This is a simple practice to stretch and strengthen the lower back and will help you to connect with the muscles of the abdomen and the pelvic floor. To begin, come to lie on your back with your knees bent about hip-width apart. You might like to use a folded blanket under your head for comfort. This starting position is known as *neutral* (figure 1 on p107), where you can notice the natural curve in the lower back. Next, keeping your buttocks on the floor, begin to create a *gentle* arch in your lower back (lumbar spine) by allowing your tailbone (coccyx) to move downward to the floor as the pelvis tilts forward. Be careful to avoid overarching the lower back. This movement is called a *pelvic tilt* (figure 2 on p107). When you are ready, keep the rest of your body relaxed and gently engage your lower belly muscles by drawing your naval to your spine and pressing your lower back into the floor, lifting the tailbone slightly. This movement is called a *pelvic thrust* (figure 3 on p107).

If each movement feels comfortable for you, begin to link the movements by moving into the pelvic tilt and then into the pelvic thrust. Find a comfortable rhythm. Then you can try to link the movements with your breath. Inhale as you move into the pelvic tilt, creating a gentle arch in the lower back and softening the belly. Exhale as you hug the belly button to your spine and flatten the lower back into the ground for the pelvic thrust. Finally, you can incorporate the muscles of your pelvic floor by engaging or lifting them on the exhale with the pelvic thrust and releasing your pelvic floor on the inhale. Repeat this sequence about 10 times and notice if you feel more of a connection to your core and pelvic floor.

If you feel any discomfort in your lower back when you move in either direction, you can leave out that part of the movement and try to move from the starting, or neutral, position into either the pelvic tilt or thrust – whichever feels more comfortable for you. Stop the practice if you feel any pain.

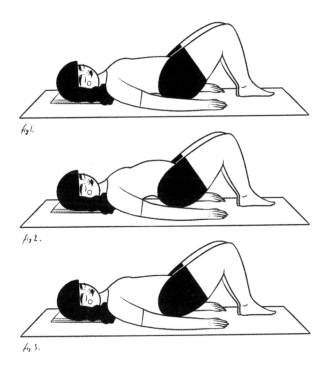

fig 1.

fig 2.

fig 3.

Letting the body be the guru

Once a foundation of embodiment has been established, you may feel more confident to trust your intuitive movement. Feeling safe in our bodies, we realise we no longer need outside teachers or validation. Letting go of the dependency on a teacher and the very rigid boundaries of some yoga lineages or traditions, you can start trusting the wisdom of the body to guide you to move in a way that feels useful. Everything that we need to be in a healthy, positive relationship with our body is within us. When we are ready, our body will start to tell us exactly how it wants to move. The body becomes the guru. It requires the mind to quieten so that the intelligence of the body can lead the movements. Like in a moving meditation, we surrender to the inner wisdom, and the body moves us in a creative dance. When we are no longer wondering what the movement looks like, what it means, or what it is doing to the muscles, all analysis is released, and we trust our body to be our ultimate guide and allow it to move us intuitively.

This practice is deeply personal. It is a chance to let go of inhibitions, and can feel sacred, spiritual and sensual. The body, mind and spirit are working in harmony as we tune into an inner wisdom deep within us. We place conscious awareness on the internal experience, that is, how the movement *feels* rather than how it *looks*. There is no expectation or goal. It is a chance to not take ourselves too seriously. We can laugh at ourselves and take pleasure in the movement. The body will know when it has moved enough, and the movement will naturally come to an end. Intuitive movement is a very simple process that leads to long-lasting transformation. Once we feel free in our body, anything is possible. All we need in order to begin is a belief in the wisdom of the body.

Intuitive movement helps us to trust ourselves

By allowing the body to guide us, we build up trust and confidence in our inner power, which is always directing us for our higher good. If we cannot trust our intuition to simply guide our movement, how can we trust it to guide us on important life decisions? Trust is like a muscle that we build up with practice. When we become overly reliant on outside experts or teachers, we hand our power to them, and we are giving ourselves a message that they know our bodies better than we do. I always tell my group yoga classes that the most advanced students are not the ones that can do the most advanced poses, but the ones who ignore me and listen to their own bodies. I love when I see people moving intuitively in class, giving their body what they need. They are connected to the wisdom of their body.

However, if we are disconnected from the wisdom of the body, we may miss the early signs that the body is communicating to get our attention when problems are developing. When we are in tune with our bodies, nobody knows our body better than us, and we trust ourselves to know when things feel different. We are then better able to communicate this internal wisdom to health professionals if we feel something is out of balance. Sometimes this might mean using our intuition to get a second, third or fourth opinion. This may be more pertinent during midlife, when we experience symptoms of hormonal decline that not all doctors are equally trained to prescribe for and support. Louann Brizendine explains that although she had medical training as a clinical psychiatrist, it wasn't until her own transition to midlife that she realised the lack of knowledge among many doctors around the symptoms women experience.[2] Trusting the intuitive intelligence of the body gives us agency and empowers us to find health professionals that can fully support us and meet our needs.

Becoming friends with the body

To take care of the body involves small right actions and slight changes in our lifestyle. This does not have to be overwhelming, and we can get help and therapeutic support to develop our connection and relationship with our body. In the first instance, slowing down to notice our relationship to our body will help. Notice how we mentally talk to our body. What language do we use? Do we hold our body in positive regard?

As we have seen, the body responds to our beliefs. All the words we tell ourselves and the words that we hear and receive from others are processed in the body, as little activations of the nervous system impacting our biochemistry. When we think negatively about ourselves, our body reacts. If we can show our bodies more love, then the body can feel this and the systems in the body can relax. This is when growth and repair can happen. When we look at our body as though it is never enough – never thin enough, never toned enough, never pretty enough, too tall, too short – whatever the specific negative self-talk we engage in, the body is always listening and responding. Hating the body, we go to war with ourselves, and we are the only looser. How we relate to our body will influence how we relate to others in our life. If we are hard on ourselves, then we are hard on others around us. And critically, how we relate to our body teaches our children how to relate to theirs. Our relationship to our body may be inherited from our parents or ancestors, and if we don't break the cycle, we may unknowingly pass damaging patterns on to our children.

The most important relationship we will have is with ourselves

As women, we heavily critique our bodies to the point where we block ourselves from believing the body has any worth or any wisdom to give us. How can we expect to be able to hear and trust our bodies when we are full of disgust for our own bodies? We must become friends with our body to deepen our ability to be intuitive to the wisdom within. If we can become aware of what is stopping us from being in the right relationship with our bodies, then we can start our healing journey.

This work of self-acceptance, love and compassion can be the work of a lifetime. Wise movement creates the conditions that help to bring us into the right relationship with our body. As we move and connect to the body, we start to feel more comfortable in our own skin. We have more vitality, and we start to enjoy our body. By becoming friends with the body, we can go deeper within, getting to know other layers of our being and allowing the conditions for wise listening. We can let go of all the harsh disapproval that we direct at ourselves and invite more softness in, watching how the world changes around us.

PRACTICE: Intuitive dancing

We each have this amazing, subtle but profound potential to connect with the wisdom of the body but, as I have mentioned earlier in relation to our inner potential, we inhibit ourselves through self-criticism, shame, guilt, lack of self-worth, embarrassment, fear and worry about what others will think. Wise intuitive movement helps us to release our inhibitions and become more confident in our bodies. Dancing alone in a safe space is a great starting point to consciously connect with the intuitive wisdom of the body. Find a time when you feel comfortable and safe in a space on your own where you won't be disturbed. Consider wearing some comfortable, loose clothes that don't feel restrictive. Put on some music that resonates with you and allow your body to move to the rhythm of the music. Aim for two to five minutes, but if you feel comfortable and the practice is enjoyable, continue for as long as you want. When you have finished, sit or lie down for one to two minutes if possible and notice how you feel.

Pearls of wisdom

○ Movement can be therapeutic, helping us to come home to our bodies and to meet ourselves in the present moment.

○ Movement can help us to safely release and let go of what the body is holding.

○ Movement creates space for the breath and circulates energy in the body.

○ Moving wisely can give us more vitality and alleviate some of the symptoms of the ageing process.

○ Movement regulates our emotions and brings us into balance.

○ Intuitive movement helps us to trust ourselves and can bring us into the right relationship with our body.

CHAPTER FIVE

Nurturing Our Energy

"*If I am not good to myself, how can I expect anyone else to be good to me?*"

MAYA ANGELOU

By practising menstrual cycle awareness, I have come to know that my energy levels fluctuate with my cycle, and that after ovulation, as my body prepares to bleed, I need to retreat and rest. And now in my forties, as I experience perimenopause, the shifting hormones compound my tiredness, and my inner wild woman rises up to fight for her needs to be met. If I don't manage my energy, the same pattern emerges every month. For a couple of days, I become an angry monster, the mother and partner I don't want to be, nagging, irritable and impatient. I become resentful of everything that I have to do, blaming my husband and kids and focusing only on household chores they haven't done rather than everything they have each contributed. I know that if I don't make time for rest and expressly ask for the support I need, the same arguments will continue to happen every month with those who live with me.

Energy awareness is crucial for our well-being in midlife. If we ignore our energetic reserves, we become depleted, running on empty, and this can eventually lead to chronic illness or burnout. In order to thrive, we must wisely tune into the natural rhythm of our energy. Conscious awareness helps us to manage and conserve this vital force, allowing us to show up as the best versions of ourselves with vibrancy and enthusiasm. Self-care is important now more than ever. It is impossible to be of service to others when we do not refuel our tank. Looking after our energy keeps us resourced – the more we have, the more we can give.

The internal energy crisis

Women are suffering an energy crisis, and the effects are impacting not only our well-being but our ability to stay in employment and earn a living. As women, many of us can attest to carrying much of the burden of domestic responsibilities, along with managing our careers and caring for children and ageing parents. It is unsurprising that we are now witnessing alarming rates of burnout amongst women. A 2022 survey of 5,000 women across 10 countries found that 53 per cent of women say their stress levels are higher than they were a year ago, and almost half feel burned out.[1] Importantly, this research shows that 40 per cent of women are actively seeking to leave their work because of burnout. We can use this epidemic of burnout as a catalyst to make our self-care a priority. How we direct, sustain and enhance our energy reserves will determine whether we can find meaning and purpose as we move into midlife.

At this time in our life, we are being pushed and pulled in so many directions with the weight of responsibilities. Many of the female clients I work with are looking after ageing parents, many of whom are ill and need care. These women do this alongside work and their own family and parenting responsibilities if they have children. As we overextend ourselves with the needs of others, we are left with little time to take care of our own energetic needs.

However, it is precisely at this time of great care-giving that we must prioritise our self-care to sustain us in whatever way we can. This might mean tiny pockets of time to connect with our breath, to do some mindful movement, to take a walk to clear our heads, or to simply have a nap and recharge our energy. When we give so much of ourselves to take care of those we love, we need to replenish our tank wherever possible. All too often, we put ourselves last, feeling selfish if we take care of our needs. What we don't realise is that when we resource ourselves sufficiently, we can have a more positive impact on those we love. A wise woman takes care of herself because she knows she can be more impactful when she has energy and vitality.

CASE STUDY: Eithne was 45 years of age and
a vice president of an international banking
company managing a large team of people. Her
job was very stressful, and she often worked
long hours, with frequent transatlantic travel.
She had a daughter who was just six years old.
Her father had dementia, and for the last few
years had needed round-the-clock care. As the
only sibling living nearby, Eithne spent one
night a week and every weekend taking care
of her dad. As you can imagine, she had no
free time for herself. Her partner wanted her
to pull back her hours looking after her dad
so that they could have more time together.
Eithne said she felt guilty juggling everything,
and that she never had enough time for her
daughter, her partner or her dad. She said she
had no social life and found it hard to keep
in touch with her friends – another thing she
felt guilty about. Eithne went into menopause
in her early forties, a couple of years after she
became a mother. Her menopausal symptoms
were intense, with hot flushes, disturbed
sleep, exhaustion, a lot of joint pain and
low libido. Her doctor prescribed HRT and
suggested that yoga might also help alleviate
her symptoms. Eithne knew that the weight of
her responsibilities was causing her stress and
impacting her health. She signed up for yoga

but would cancel appointments, saying that she couldn't take the time for herself when everyone else needed her. Some weeks later, Eithne fell while walking her dog and broke her leg, and was incapacitated for almost three months. During this time, she needed help from her partner to shower and get dressed. Her friends dropped off dinners and helped with school runs. She couldn't drive and had to employ a carer to help with her dad. The experience taught her to slow down and recognise that unless she was in good health, she would not be able to be there for anyone else. At last she understood that filling her own tank was not selfish; on the contrary, it enabled her to show up and support the other people in her life. Eithne spoke to her company and was able to move to a four-day working week. She started her yoga therapy sessions on her day off, and we explored gentle movements to help strengthen her body after the injury and breathing practices to help her relax and manage stress. Along with yoga therapy, Eithne booked a block of monthly reflexology sessions that was covered by her health insurance. Having more time for herself helped her to feel more relaxed and less overwhelmed by her responsibilities.

Functional breathing

The first step in wisely managing our reserves is understanding how energy sustains our well-being. As I mentioned previously, we take in vital energy or life force from the universe through our breath, and how we breathe impacts the amount of energy we allow into our body and our biochemistry. When we are relaxed, our breath is deeper and smoother, allowing us to take in more vital energy and helping to balance the body. The stress response encourages our breathing to become rapid and shallow. This is intended only as a short-term response, and chronic stress can lead to long-term dysfunctional breathing patterns.

The simple act of noticing and training our breath can transform our lives. To breathe functionally, we inhale and exhale through the nose. It also requires that we use the diaphragm as the primary breathing muscle. When we inhale, our diaphragm engages and moves downwards, causing our belly to push out. This allows our lungs to expand. On the exhale, our diaphragm relaxes and moves back up so the belly can move back in towards the spine. This *diaphragmatic breathing* facilitates the breath in coming into the full length of the lungs. It is the most efficient way to breathe. This is also important because the undulation of the diaphragm supports the vagus nerve in switching on the relaxation response. When we do this, we signal to the body that it is safe to relax. Our heart rate slows down and our blood pressure drops. That is why deep belly breaths have a calming and soothing effect.

As women, we have been culturally conditioned to make our bellies appear smaller. We can often hold a lot of tension and tightness in the area of the abdomen, and it may not feel easy to soften the belly to allow the diaphragm to move in the way it needs to with our breath. This can be even more difficult if we have had surgery such as caesarean deliveries or a hysterectomy, as we can be unconsciously protecting scar tissue that may actually benefit from gentle stretching. Some of us are *reverse breathers* – meaning that when we inhale we pull the belly in and when we exhale we push the belly out. Reverse breathing is a dysfunctional breathing pattern that stops us from receiving optimal energy from the breath. We might also be *chest breathers*. This results in a shallow breath in the upper lungs and an overreliance on the secondary breathing muscles, which are in the chest, neck and shoulders. Often this leads to chronic tightness in those muscles, which can be the root cause of tension in that area of the body.

PRACTICE: Breath awareness

This short breathing practice will help you to become more aware of how you breathe. Begin by sitting or lying down comfortably. (If you like, you can bend the knees to relieve any lower back pain.) When you are ready, just start to breathe naturally. Notice if you are breathing through the nose or the mouth. If you find that you are mouth breathing, see if it is possible to breathe in and out through the nose.

If this is uncomfortable for you, don't worry — please just breathe naturally.

Start to notice the *rhythm* of your breath. For example, are you breathing fast or slowly? Shallow or deep? Notice if there is anywhere in your body where you can feel the breath. Do you feel it in your neck, shoulders or chest? Or maybe down towards your ribs or your belly? Can you notice if the front body is rising when you inhale and falling when you exhale? Now, see if it is possible for you to consciously soften your abdomen, just allowing the whole belly to completely relax. If it's useful, you can place the hands on the belly. Allow the inhale to come down towards the belly. Do you feel the belly rise on the inhale and fall on the exhale? Or the other way around? Take a few slow, smooth breaths. Just follow the movement of the belly as you breathe. If you are comfortable here, you may want to count the length of your inhale and the length of your exhale. Notice the ratio of your breath (for example, if the inhale is 4 and the exhale is 6, the ratio is 4:6). After a few moments, just allow your breath to come back to your own natural rhythm. You may want to reflect on the following questions to help you get to know your own breathing patterns:

○ Are you naturally breathing through your mouth or your nose?

○ Where in the body could you feel the breath?

○ Did your breathing feel shallow or deep?

○ Do you reverse breathe, holding the belly in on the inhale and pushing out on the exhale?

○ Which part of the breath feels easier – the inhale or the exhale? If the inhale felt easier, do you feel like you are able to fully exhale or do you hold your breath?

○ Was your exhale longer than your inhale?

○ Did you notice any effects on your mind after working with your breath? Did you feel more relaxed or anxious?

Yoga and the breath

Please don't worry if this was difficult for you. It can take some time to change our habitual breathing patterns. But we can train our breath with practice. When we breathe functionally, we take in enough energy to oxygenate the systems of the body, fueling our health. In yoga, we focus on lengthening the exhale to help us release the old before we welcome in the new. The inhale comes after the exhale.

Dysfunctional breathing patterns impact not only our physiological health but also our psychological health. When we don't feel like we have enough breath, we can feel anxious and distressed, and this can result in panic attacks or hyperventilation.

The ancient yogis believed that we each have a certain number of breaths allocated to our life. They focused on breathing slower and deeper to prolong life. The Hindu scripture the *Bhagavad Gita* says we should be inspired to live like the tortoise.[2] The tortoise has a slow breathing rate of three to four breaths per minute and can live to between 250 and 300 years. When we take slower, deeper breaths in and out through the nose, we lower our heart rate, activate the relaxation response, and bring ourselves into the present moment, conserving our energy, enhancing our vitality and perhaps improving our longevity.

The seven chakras

In my work as a yoga therapist and a reiki practitioner, I am concerned with the subtle energy field of the body. These healing modalities identify seven main energy centres in our body called the *chakras* – with *chakra* meaning wheel. Each chakra is a vortex of energy that expresses a different physical, emotional, creative and spiritual component. The chakras run from just above the crown of the head down to the tailbone and they map onto the major glands of the endocrine system, which produce our hormones. In energy healing, we use hand positions and sacred symbols to help the vital life force, *reiki* or *prana*, to flow through the chakras. In yoga, we use movement with the breath to encourage the flow of energy through the chakras. The chakras can be visualised as spinning wheels of light.

1. Crown chakra: This is located just above the crown of our head and relates to our whole being and our sense of connection to the whole of life. It is our link with the universe and a higher power. This chakra maps onto the pineal gland. The energy of the crown chakra is represented by the colours violet or white.

2. Forehead chakra: This is located at the third eye in between the eyebrows. It governs the brain, the eyes and the sinuses. This maps onto the pituitary gland. This energy centre relates to intuition, clarity and insight and to our spiritual connection. The energy of the third eye is represented by the colour indigo.

3. Throat chakra: Located at the centre of the throat, this governs our mouth, jaw, thyroid, neck and shoulders. This maps onto the thyroid gland. It relates to our self-expression, speech and communication, and whether we can speak our truth. We block our throat chakra when we don't express how we feel or what we want to say. The energy of the throat is represented by the colour blue.

4. Heart chakra: This connects our higher and lower chakras. It governs the heart, chest, lungs, arms and hands. This maps onto the thymus gland. It is related to love. When the heart chakra is open, we can allow love in and out. To protect ourselves from pain, sometimes we close the heart and cut ourselves off from others. When we open our heart to all that we can experience and feel in life, we come to know that to experience

love and joy we must also experience pain and suffering. The energy of the heart is represented by the colours green or pink.

5. Solar plexus chakra: This is located just above the navel and below the ribcage. It governs digestion, the stomach, the small intestine, the liver, the gall bladder and the spleen. This maps onto the digestive gland, the pancreas. It is connected to our identity within our communities and our seat of wisdom and power, and to our ability to take action with our creativity. It is represented by the colour yellow.

6. Sacral chakra: This is located at the centre of the pelvis. It relates to the reproductive organs, the bladder and the kidneys. This maps onto our adrenal glands. It is our centre of balance, playfulness, sexuality and creativity. Sacral energy is represented by the colour orange.

7. Root chakra: This is located at the base of the spine, at the tailbone. It governs our large intestine, rectum, legs and feet. This maps onto the gonads or sex glands – the ovaries in women and the testes in men. It is our connection to the earth and our sense of trust. The root is related to our basic survival and determines if we sense fear or safety in the world. If the root chakra is open, we feel supported by life. The energy of the root is represented by the colour red.

THE SEVEN CHAKRAS

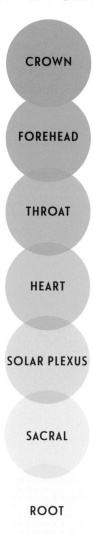

CROWN

FOREHEAD

THROAT

HEART

SOLAR PLEXUS

SACRAL

ROOT

The five winds of energy

Along with the energy centres, the direction or flow of energy is important for our vitality. Yoga speaks of five *vayus*, meaning winds of energy, which are currents of energy responsible for transporting life force through channels or nadis to the different chakras, glands, organs, cells, tissues, bones and empty spaces in the body. The five vayus are:

1. Prana vayu: This governs the heart, chest and head. The direction of this energy is inwards and upwards. On the physical level, it is responsible for breathing, eating, drinking and swallowing. It also relates to how we take in information and experiences and move forward in our life. Prana is weakened by sensory overload. It is strengthened with silence and focusing inwards. When prana vayu is weak, the mind cannot focus.

2. Apana vayu: This is located in the pelvis. It is responsible for elimination. The direction of this energy is down and out. It relates to our ability to let go of difficult thoughts or feelings. When apana is healthy, we can experience difficulty, process it, and then release it. If apana is weak, our mind is full of worries and we may feel ungrounded and unsupported.

3. Samana vayu: This is located at the navel and is a circular movement. It governs digestion, assimilation and how we absorb things in the body. It is related to our gut instinct. When samana is weak or blocked, we can experience digestive problems, feelings of depletion

and an inability to think and talk about difficult experiences. If samana is strong, we can see difficulties as opportunities for learning and growth, and we can easily let go of any negativity that might weigh us down.

4. Udana vayu: This is located at the throat and governs speech, expression and ascension. It is an upward movement. It is responsible for growth and our ability to reach beyond limitations. If udana is weak, we can feel stagnant and lack enthusiasm in our life. We may also feel unable to speak up and express our needs.

5. Vyana vayu: This governs the whole body. It is responsible for the circulation of food, water and oxygen. It also determines the circulation of ideas, thoughts and emotions. When vyana is healthy, we can express ourselves in a loving way and feel fearless and outgoing. Inefficient vyana can lead to isolation, separation and alienation, and it can limit our beliefs, thoughts or emotions.

As we transition to midlife, we must manage our inner energy wisely to keep us vibrant, inspired and enthused. When our chakras are balanced and the vayus are functioning, the energy is freely flowing through the spine and central nervous system and out into the rest of the body and the peripheral nervous system. When the energy is flowing easily, the inner organs receive sufficient life force to function well. By working with our breath and moving with intuitive wisdom, we influence our vitality and support the natural flow within the subtle energy body, invigorating every layer of our being.

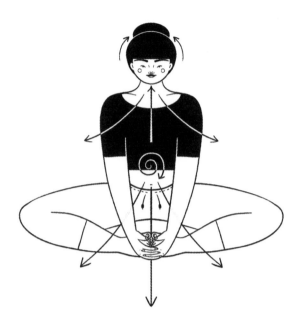

Refuelling with nutrition

We need to consciously cultivate the right conditions to resource ourselves energetically. As we deepen our connection to our inner self, our awareness expands, and we may start to notice how we feel after certain foods. This can help us to be more discerning and choose the right food to nourish us. The food we eat fuels our body and impacts our gut health. During midlife, changing hormone levels can affect our blood sugar, causing spikes or crashes. These can also be exacerbated by stress hormones.

Midlife is an important time to consider our relationship with food. We can influence our energy and overall well-being by the foods we choose to nourish us.

If in the past, like me, you have had a complex relationship with food, midlife might see some of those issues re-emerge. My perimenopause affected my blood sugar, and I had intense sugar cravings. I began to forgo meals for chocolate, making my sugar imbalance worse and triggering my old patterns of disordered eating. My gut was irritated from all the chocolate affecting my enteric nervous system. I had pangs of sadness and anxiety in my gut that I never had before.

Getting curious about the relationship between food and mood helped me to come back into balance. I started to introduce protein at every meal to stabilise my blood sugar, and I increased my intake of oestrogen-boosting foods like soy and flaxseeds. To help heal my gut, I ate miso, kefir and live probiotic yogurt. However, as I mentioned earlier, I have had a complex relationship with food, and nutrition is beyond my scope of practice as a yoga therapist. We are all different, and what works for one person might not work for another. So when I share my experience, it is only to encourage you to consider how your food choices might support your physical, mental and emotional health during your transition to midlife. Those of us who have had a challenging relationship with food or who have suffered from an eating disorder can use this time in our lives to seek out therapeutic support to finally heal this part of ourselves and allow food the opportunity to repair and nourish our well-being and give us the energy that we need.

Eating in rhythm with the seasons

Many of us are detached from the cycles of nature, but eating seasonally provides us with an abundance of produce that contains timely vitamins and minerals for that time of year. Masanobu Fukuoka was a farmer in Japan who advocated a return to natural farming methods. His enlightening book *The One-Straw Revolution* demonstrates how many of our problems stem from our disconnection with nature and with where our food comes from. He said that 'food is life, and life must not step away from nature'.[3] There is no perfect diet, and as I know only too well, we can become disordered in our eating habits if we strive to eat perfectly. But if we can choose simple, local, seasonal produce that is wholesome and flavoursome, we receive more life-force energy.

We also have an emotional relationship with food. Marc David, the author of *Nourishing Wisdom*, says that 'you are what you eat, and you eat what you are'.[4] He suggests that how we think and feel about ourselves will determine the types of food we reach for. Furthermore, he said that if we eat with the mindset of guilt or shame around our food, then this will influence how our body digests and assimilates food. Attuning to our inner wisdom, we can eat with the natural rhythm of the body and enjoy our food. Slowing down to take time to plan and prepare our food in sync with the seasons will serve our energy.

Our digital diet

The content we feed the mind through our digital diet, the media we consume, the music we listen to, the books we read and the movies we watch can all influence the quality of our thoughts and, in turn, our energy. Notice how you feel the next time you spend a bit of time scrolling through your newsfeed. Consider if the consumption of this content moves you towards fear or towards love. As we know from our discussion of the nervous system, fear-based thoughts and beliefs create stress on our system, diminishing our energy, whereas love moves us towards growth and replenishment.

Sleep – the great reset

We need about eight hours of sleep per night. Sleep is the great reset button, when the nervous system can heal, restore and come back into balance. In a state of chronic fatigue, our energetic reserves are depleted, putting our physical body under stress. Our reactions and responses are more emotionally charged because we have not had enough time to refuel.

One common symptom in perimenopause, as the hormones shift and change, is disturbed sleep. Women also often describe feeling an increase in anger and rage as they transition to midlife. These emotions can arise from the stress hormones released through exhaustion and lack of sleep. We become overwhelmed and frustrated when we don't prioritise our own energetic needs. Sometimes we revel in the self-sacrifices we make for others, becoming martyrs, only to implode or explode with resentment. We might argue with our family, blaming them for putting demands on our energy. But as wise women, we must recognise that we are responsible for carving out sacred time to replenish and prevent burnout. We cannot wait for others to offer us opportunities to recharge. We must give ourselves permission to respond to our needs first, because we cannot give what we don't have.

CASE STUDY: When Nina came to see me, she was sleeping only two hours a night. She was a mum with a fulltime job and had a large family. Although she had read up on perimenopause and was aware that her sleep disturbance could be a result of hormones, it took her two years before she sought support and medical advice. Her life was so busy taking care of everyone else that she didn't prioritise her own needs. She was muddling through on an empty tank. By taking time for herself and practising yoga, and with the right cocktail of HRT, her sleep started to improve. She still doesn't get the full optimum seven–nine hours' sleep, but she is getting a lot more than before she started to take care of herself.

Yoga nidra for deep rest

Yoga nidra is a practice of deep relaxation that we can use to replenish our energy or to help us to relax and prepare for sleep. The practice allows us to reach the hypnagogic state, which is the point between waking and sleeping. Many people fall asleep when they first start the practice. Over time, you might be able to follow the guidance and stay awake, just drifting in and out. If you think you might fall sleep, you can set an alarm to wake you up. Yoga nidra can be used as a little siesta or can be practised any time you feel like you need to recharge to have more energy for your day. It is especially useful after lunch to aid digestion – which can only happen when we are relaxed – or to cope with the afternoon lull that often happens around four o'clock. You can also practise it just before bed to help prepare for sleep.

PRACTICE: 61-points yoga nidra

There are many types of yoga nidra. The practice I offer here is called 61 points and it takes about 12 to 15 minutes. It is a guided body scan that includes awareness of most of the energy centres, or chakras, of the body. It is suitable for most people, though if you currently don't find it is safe to relax during the short, silent pauses, you are welcome to leave the pauses out, or leave the practice out altogether. Whenever you do feel comfortable to try it, you could record yourself

reading the practice aloud and then play it to yourself.
To begin, come to lie comfortably on your back, either on
a bed, on a couch or on the floor. You might like to place
a pillow under your knees to support your lower back and
put something soft under your head. Cover yourself with a
blanket to keep warm. Make any little adjustments you need
to feel as comfortable as possible. When you are ready, you
might like to close the eyes.

Allow the body to soften to the support of the earth
beneath you. Feel the earth holding you. Begin to notice
the sounds around you and gently let the sounds wash
over you, letting go of attachment to sound. When you are
ready, start to notice your body breathing. Sense the belly
rising and falling with each breath. As you inhale, the belly
rises slightly, and as you exhale, the belly relaxes. Have
the intention that the place you are in is a safe, nurturing
and healing space. You can relax here safely. Slowly allow
the breath to deepen. Know that the inhale is a nourishing,
healing breath, while the exhale is a chance to release and
let go. Begin to invite the whole body to soften, letting go
of all tension or tightness. As the body relaxes, the breath
becomes very gentle.

Begin to witness the body breathing now without any
conscious effort. Now let the awareness come to the point
between the eyebrows, also known as the third eye chakra.

Feel or imagine a point of light here. Relax the whole body.
Now the awareness moves to the throat chakra. In your
mind's eye, see a point of light at the centre of the throat.
The whole body is resting. Now the tip of the right shoulder
joint, a point of light. Right elbow. Right wrist. Tip of the right
thumb, a point of light. The index finger, middle finger, ring
finger, the little finger, a point of light. Now the centre of the
right wrist. Right elbow joint. Right shoulder. Relax. Throat
centre. Left shoulder, a point of light. Left elbow. Centre of
the left wrist. Tip of left thumb, index finger, middle finger,
ring finger, little finger. Centre of left wrist. Left elbow joint.
Left shoulder. Centre of throat. Heart centre. Right chest
or breast. Heart centre. Left chest or breast, a point of light.
Heart centre. Navel centre just below the ribs. Now centre
of the pelvis. Centre of right hip. Right knee. Right ankle.
Tip of the big toe, second toe, third toe, fourth toe, little toe.
Centre of right ankle. Right knee. Right hip. Centre of pelvis.
Left hip. Left knee. Left ankle. Big toe, second toe, third toe,
fourth toe, little toe. Centre of left ankle. Left knee. Centre of
left hip. Centre of pelvis. Navel centre. Heart centre. Throat
centre. Point between the eyebrows, a point of light. Feel
the whole body spacious and open. See all of the points of
light at once. Witness these points as stars in a galaxy. Allow
yourself to deeply rest in this sense of spacious awareness.
Fully drop into this deep sense of peace.

(Two-minute pause.)

Then, slowly begin to come back to the breath. Start to allow the breath to come into the body a little deeper now. When you are ready, slowly begin to bring a little bit of gentle movement to the fingers and the toes. Taking your time, slowly roll over onto your side. Take a moment to notice how you feel. Then gradually think about gently coming back to sit.

We are all connected energetically

We are each part of a universal energetic field. Our inner energy is interacting with the energy all around us. Considering that your exhale becomes part of my inhale and vice versa, it is hard to refute that we are all interconnected beings. We absorb source energy from the macro field and release energy back into this field. Life is an energetic exchange. Everyone has their own frequency and vibration. Our thoughts, beliefs, words and actions infuse our own unique energetic vibration that shapes the macro energy field.

With this great power comes a responsibility to play our part in making the world a more harmonious, joyful and peaceful place. By sustaining and enriching our vital energy, we raise our vibration and become more useful and purposeful in the world. To be of service, we need our energy to be balanced. Therefore, our priority is to take care of our own vital energy. First, we must be aware of it so that we can start to become attuned to the warning signs that it is running low. When we are in tune with it, then we can do what needs to be done to change our energy and shift our vibration.

The dynamics of our energetic exchanges

As a vessel of energy, we receive energy in and offer energy out. Our vibrations interact with others in an energetic exchange. When our social relationships are in alignment with our energetic vibrations, we can feel safe, supported, sustained and comfortable in the company of others. Our nervous system is relaxed and the chemistry in the body is not thrown out of balance from the social interaction.

In physics, this energetic exchange is called 'constructive interference'. However, if our energy is out of alignment with the frequency of another, we may not feel secure, and our nervous system may feel threatened or stressed, activating the stress response and changing the chemical balance in our body. The quality of our thoughts may be affected, and we may feel less vitality after spending time in their company. This is known in physics as 'destructive interference'.

Depending on our sensitivity to energy, we may either be conscious or unaware of the shift in dynamics in our interactions. But it is highly likely that we have all experienced the sensation of being in the company of others and feeling either uplifted or drained. It is important to remember that just as we gain energy from others, our own vibration can deplete another person's energetic resources. How we show up in the world can activate the stress response of others. Our cultural socialisation, which creates our beliefs and attitudes towards others, will shape our energy towards them. If we have been taught to be fearful or threatened by certain people in society, then our interactions will activate the stress response in both us and them. When there is a sympathetic activation, the brain becomes more narrowly focused, less open-minded and more defensive, and we draw on old judgement patterns.

Stress energy heightens divisiveness in society. We have seen this all over the world in the last couple of years. The pandemic has been a collective trauma that has inflamed the stress response at a global level, leading to more tensions, divisions and a sense of separateness among people. Now more than ever, it is critical that we develop awareness of our own energy, becoming more mindful of our energetic exchanges to manage them in a way that creates more balance, unity and harmony in our inner and outer world. To do this, we must exercise wise discernment to come into the right rhythm with our energy. As wise women, we have the opportunity to transform how we show up in the world. We can consciously choose to be an authentic, unifying force of energy.

Wise discernment

There are times when we need to protect our energy. This requires a sense of discernment about how we spend our time and about whom we spend our time with. A sense of obligation, shame or guilt can see us return time and time again to situations and relationships that deplete our energy. Our energy maintenance depends on our ability to say no. One of the biggest threats to our vitality is what Oprah Winfrey calls 'our disease to please'.[5] As little girls, we may have been encouraged to people please, and unconsciously we can pass this on to our own children. We may tell kids to say yes when they mean no. Our actions may tell them to change who they are to make others feel comfortable. But our purpose in this world is not to change or hide the essence of who we are to make others feel comfortable. We each have an amazing potential to bring goodness into the world. But it requires the confidence to stay true to who we are and to say no if we need to.

Learning how to say no

We want our daughters to be able to say no – and to say a full yes, too, when they mean it! We wish for them to know what they want and not to repress it. But they need us to demonstrate this behaviour, so we may also need to get better at saying no. Unlike many women, my family is not dependent on my income so I can sometimes teach yoga for free. For many years, I offered free therapeutic yoga for children in special education, and it was extremely rewarding to see how yoga could benefit these amazing children. Word got around in my local area about the classes and other schools approached me to volunteer with them. My schedule was fairly full already, but I didn't want to disappoint the schools, so I agreed to take on more volunteer work. Committing to so many classes was exhausting, and without the energetic exchange of money, I felt undervalued and resentful. I needed to pull back, but I was reluctant to as I didn't want to be seen as selfish. I was wrestling with a lot of guilt over my privileged financial position, and a part of me felt that I was not worthy to use my time to earn my own money. I was bound by a sense of duty to alleviate my guilt for the abundance that I had, and this had started to overshadow my intention to volunteer. I was no longer serving the children or myself. I realised that I had to pull back and find my voice to say no to certain requests. This was the only way to find equanimity and serve others without burning out.

As well as getting better at saying no, we must also get better at respecting and allowing other women to say no. When we are used to people in our lives saying yes, we can be affronted when they say no; but by respecting the responses of others, we give ourselves more permission to honour our truth.

If we say yes when we mean no, we deny our truth. Ultimately, this can cause a lot of hurt and pain for both ourselves and others. When I was 30 years old, I said yes to a marriage proposal because I didn't know how to say no. I told myself I didn't want to hurt my boyfriend at the time. It suited me to play the martyr, excusing my behaviour as saving his feelings. But I hurt us both by not being truthful and caused myself more pain and shame when I broke off the engagement after six weeks.

It is common to blame others and play the victim when we have not expressed our truth. We internally reproach them, thinking *how could they ask me that?* or *the nerve of them.* To take the focus off us, we project it onto them, forgetting that they are entitled to ask, just as we are equally entitled to say no. We have free will and we have a choice.

The niggle of a no

It takes so much energy when we have said yes when we mean no. Then we have to figure out a way to back-track and turn our yes back into a no. And we know the sensations and the feelings in our body when we have gone against our truth, and the niggle that won't leave us until we find a solution that brings us back to our authenticity. We all know how this consumes our resources. We also all know the energy we save when we speak our truth in the first instance. Saying no might make us feel uncomfortable in the short term, but the more we honour our truth the less hurt we cause everyone around us in the long term.

We can start by practising saying small noes. This is how we develop the confidence and courage to say no in more challenging or confronting circumstances. This is part of building up our *truth muscle.* If we don't flex our truth muscle, we lose our sense of self – *use it or lose it*, as the saying goes. We become so removed from who we are that we no longer know our own truth. In my own case, dishonouring my truth and silencing my noes caused me to disassociate from my body, numb my feelings, and exile my inner guide. We use up a lot of energy, damaging ourselves, by pretending to be something we are not.

The energetic rhythm of midlife

As we move towards midlife, the hormonal waves can cause us to become less interested in people pleasing. We are no longer bathing in the summer waters of oestrogen that nature provides to help us attract a mate and reproduce. We may find that we become less tolerant of situations that we would have previously endured to please others. After living half our lives pleasing others, it is time to put our energy into pleasing ourselves without harming others. We can use our time and energy on things that make us feel enthusiastic and inspired. This is not selfish. It is nourishing and enriching our energy so that we can show up as the best version of ourselves and have something positive to offer to the world.

Only by becoming more conscious of our energy body can we notice what invigorates and lights us up. When we know how we lose energy through our lifestyle, actions, behaviours or relationships, we can make changes to refuel and replenish our resources. We can give and we can take in balance and harmony with the universal energy field. Living in the right rhythm, we are of course naturally ageing, but we are not old or redundant. We can still be young at heart, open to new ideas, continually learning, creating and expressing ourselves in new ways. We can get to choose to use our energy wisely. We have free will to decide this. Do we give it all away, or do we nourish ourselves and come into a wise rhythm, expressing our energy intelligently, creatively and purposefully? Choosing the latter, we can move into midlife bursting with vibrancy, meaning and purpose. Of course, it is important to acknowledge that this is easier for some of us than for others, and may be influenced by our geography, by our personal circumstances and experiences, and by our underlying physical and mental health.

PRACTICE: The pause

We are living in a world where we are now overly accessible to requests 24 hours a day through our smartphone. Every request demands our energetic attention and invites a flurry of emotions and thoughts. When we feel pressure to respond immediately, our reactions are rushed and pressurised. This is dangerous ground for people pleasers, who find it hard to say no. When we give ourselves permission to take our time to respond, we can prevent ourselves from overcommitting our time and saying yes when we mean no.

Try this simple tip of delaying your responses. When you receive a request for your energy, take time for contemplation and reflection. Meditate on the request. Tune into your internal feelings and see how the request sits with you. Notice if the request triggers something in you. Ask yourself how you would respond if you were being true to your authentic self. If saying no causes you worry and anxiety, it may help to write down your feelings to help you process them. Take a few moments to connect with your breath to bring you into the present moment and develop a sense of calm. Ask yourself if you need more time to think about it. Only respond to the request when you feel calm, grounded and centred and are able to answer in a way that is true for you. It may take a few hours or even a couple of days or weeks until you are ready to respond. You may like to note your response and how your feel after you have replied. Record the outcome in a journal or diary. This way, you can refer back to it the next time a difficult request comes up.

Pearls of wisdom

- We can be more impactful when we have energy and vitality.
- Functional breathing gives us more energy and calms our nervous system.
- We can fuel ourselves with right nutrition, a positive relationship with food and plenty of rest and sleep.
- We are all connected energetically, and we influence each other by how we show up in the world.
- We get to choose how to use our energy wisely, and sometimes we have to say no to sustain our energy.

CHAPTER SIX

Finding Clarity

"Where our attention goes, our energy flows"

SHAUNA SHAPIRO

To become a truth-teller in midlife, we must find clarity of thought. The mind can tell us a story that is simply not true. And as we journey inwards, we must get to know the intricacies of our thoughts, becoming aware of what causes us mental disturbances and learning to distinguish between the fact and fiction in our heads. No matter what practices we do, if our thoughts continue to deceive us, we will be unable to see clearly and access our true power in midlife.

The power of our thoughts

To use our energy wisely, we must get to know our mind, as it plays a chief role in sustaining or draining our energy. How and what we think creates a sense of either safety or threat, which we know changes the chemistry in the body, activating either the relaxation response or the stress response.

Within our limbic or emotional brain, which is responsible for monitoring danger, we have an almond-shaped fire alarm called the amygdala. When we experience a real or perceived threat, it is our amygdala that goes on high alert, sounding the fire alarm to the rest of the body to activate the stress response. Our thoughts have the power to hijack the amygdala and sound the alarm. Once the alarm has been sounded, it overwhelms our rational brain, called the cortex, and we become dysregulated, or unable to control our emotional reactions. Important higher executive functions of the brain responsible for language, rational thought, imagination, consciousness, learning, choice, empathy and awareness of self are all overridden once this fire alarm goes off.

I have a fear of flying, and my amygdala sounds the fire alarm in my brain every time I am on an aeroplane. Once there is a bit of turbulence, very quickly my thoughts become negative and I find myself consumed by the thought of death. Even though I know rationally that turbulence is normal and that the pilot is highly skilled to deal with it, when I am on the flight my amygdala takes over and I am no longer in my rational brain. My brain responds to my fear by activating the stress response and flooding my body with stress hormones. When this happens, I always do my best to practise deep belly breathing to activate my vagus nerve, which would normally stimulate the parasympathetic nervous system and calm me down. But unless I change my thinking and stop sending the message to my brain that I am in danger, I am unable to calm my nervous system down. This is the power that we can give our thoughts.

What if the thoughts are not true?

If you don't share this fear of flying, my response may seem like a complete overreaction. But perhaps you have experienced this reaction in your own body from your own fearful thoughts, phobias or memory of trauma. Once we give enough momentum to our fearful thoughts, they sound our amygdala alarm and hijack our responses. It therefore follows that we only want this alarm to go off with good reason! However, what we think is often not a true reflection of reality. Our brain naturally defaults to negative thinking. This is what happens to me on a flight – my mind defaults to *thinking* the worst in an effort to *prepare* me for the worst. This is how we are programmed for survival. And because of this bias towards the negative, the mind does not always speak the truth – it can be our best friend and our worst enemy.

What is behind our thoughts?

To find clarity and insight, it is really important for us to take our own thoughts with a pinch of salt and to get curious about whether they are motivated by fear or truth. Our thoughts are energetic fluctuations that arise from our feelings, emotions, beliefs and attitudes. Everything we think is shaped by preconceived judgements and biases that we hold about ourselves and others. These judgements and biases are influenced by cultural and social norms and by familial and individual life experiences. We may be unconsciously aware of many of these biases, but they can be at the root of much of our fear-based thinking. They drive our behaviours and are responsible for many divisions in society.

Our unconscious biases are behind our many prejudices towards our fellow humans. Historically, we have been conditioned to live in fear of people who are different from us, and this fear is strengthened when we live in communities that lack diversity. If we come from a homogeneous community and are constantly surrounded only by people who look like us, act like us and live like us, then when we leave our community and encounter more diversity we can feel threatened, and our fears will activate the stress response.

I moved to London from a small town in Ireland, and despite travelling abroad and going to university in Dublin city, up until that point I had only ever had one Black friend and one Asian friend. Living and working in a multicultural city like London was a learning experience for me, heightening my awareness of biases that I never even knew I had and which I definitely did not want to admit to having. Whether we want to admit it or not, we all have unconscious biases from our familial, social and cultural conditioning. Rather than ignoring them or pretending they don't exist, we must begin to shine a light of awareness on our unconscious biases and acknowledge the role they play in our thoughts and decisions, so that we can work towards shifting them for the greater good.

CASE STUDY: Ann-Marie was 46 years old, a mother of four who lived in a suburban town on the outskirts of Dublin. She was active on the parents' committee at her children's school and she fundraised regularly for local charities. Both she and her husband had worked hard to be able to afford a house in an affluent area, near a nice park that the kids enjoyed visiting most days after school. Just as they finished a major renovation on the house, rumours began to spread around the neighbourhood that the local council had agreed to the establishment of a homeless shelter for drug users on the same street where Ann-Marie lived. Many of the neighbours began to get concerned and organised a meeting. They spoke about their fears about what this might mean for the safety of their street, and they organised a petition to stop the centre from going ahead without their consultation. Ann-Marie started to become afraid. She worried that the shelter would lead to an increase in anti-social behaviour and that she would no longer feel safe in her dream home. She felt that the shelter would devalue house prices on the street and that the park would no longer be a safe place for her children to play in. When she spoke to me about her concerns, I could see that her amygdala was firing the alarm at the very thought of the centre.

Knowing her to be very kind and giving,
I suggested that her thoughts might be coming
from a place of fear and uncertainty. All of her
worries were based in the future, and she was
assuming that the centre would have a negative
impact on her street. I asked her to take a few
moments to consider her unconscious biases
towards the potential clients of the homeless
shelter. Could she see that she was basing her
prejudgements on negative stereotypes without
knowing these people? Could she allow herself
to see that the clients who needed the centre
were just like her and me, but that maybe they
had faced more suffering in their lives? I asked
her if she could consider that her reaction to
the centre was an opportunity to teach her
children the values she wanted to try to instil
in them. By allowing fear to take charge of
her reaction, she was teaching her children to
fear people who might live a different life to
them. Could she choose to consider that the
centre might actually have a positive impact
on the community, and that it could be an
opportunity to teach her children empathy and
understanding for others? When she took a
step back from her thoughts, Ann-Marie could
see that her reaction was based on fear. She
decided not to sign the petition objecting to
the shelter. When it finally did open, she met

with the manager to find out more about the
work. Ann-Marie learned that the shelter
worked closely with the local police station
to prevent anti-social behaviour and to keep
the park a safe place for all the local children.
Inspired by what she saw, she asked if she
could use her skills to help with fundraising for
resources for the shelter.

Do we want an individualistic or a collective culture?

Millions of people today don't feel safe in their body, in
their environment and in our society. Many are facing bat-
tles to be accepted by others. The current global media
culture intensifies a sense of danger and mistrust within
each of us. And the narrative of 'every person for themselves' thrives in this fear-based climate, resulting in the
individualistic society we have today, with a culture that
prioritises individual needs over the needs of the whole
community. In our world, success is defined in terms of
profit and financial gain, often achieved at any cost.

We have witnessed how this type of society continues
to damage our environment, divide our communities
and cause untold trauma, pain and suffering. History
has given us all the ancestral legacy of colonialism, gen-
ocide, racism, slavery, sexism, classism, ableism, ageism,
homophobia and stigma. Currently, a multitude of abuses
of power continue throughout the world, dominating

and dividing people so that others can benefit and exploit resources for themselves. Whether the system has privileged or discriminated against us personally, it has left an imprint on all of us, and healing and transforming our shared collective pain and trauma begins with recognition. Our past may have been rooted in fear, scarcity and lack, but there is another way to live, whereby we expand our circle of love beyond our individual families and friends into the wider community, the country and the world. Now, more than ever, we need a society that is more unified than fractured – based on a sense of belonging and connection. To come together, we need to feel safe enough at the individual level to trust that collectively we can create changes that support all of us and our planet.

How does our individual mindset influence our worldview?

Our individual mindset influences how we view the world and what we allow into our life. If we view the world through a lens of *scarcity*, we believe that there are not enough resources and opportunities to go around. We are driven by fear, competition and a sense of lack, and we think another person's successes, achievements and level of happiness leave a lesser share for us. We become attached to our possessions, clinging to them, frightened of losing what we do have, and becoming threatened by the lives of others.

This mindset is underpinned by fear, resulting in a chronic stress response in our bodies. However, if we can shift our worldview to look through the lens of *abundance*, we can see that the universe has unlimited opportunities. With this mindset, we are not threatened by another's happiness, successes, achievements and gains, as we know they do not diminish the chance we have to obtain these for ourselves. Believing in universal abundance, we are genuinely grateful and relish in the success of others, because their success does not mean that there are fewer resources available to us. While a scarcity mindset originates from fear, an abundance mindset is rooted in love and consequently results in a more relaxed nervous system.

How do we shift our mindset towards abundance?

Some of the wisest work we can do now is to become aware of our mindset and reduce the impressions of lack and scarcity. Given cultural norms and the legacy of the past, fear and scarcity are deeply entrenched in many people's psyche. This mindset is energised every time we turn on the news. With every bad news story, our amygdala sets off the fire alarm and the cycle begins again. The medicine for our global nervous system is love. Positive experiences feed the prefrontal cortex in the brain, reducing the stress response. Bringing more love and joy into our lives calms our nervous system. Pleasure is both medicinal and our birthright, but our burnout culture has forgotten this. We must cast off our old ways of thinking and find a sense of tranquillity to allow ourselves to return to love.

Nourishing the seeds of contentment

Neuroscience shows that expressing gratitude changes the structures in our brain and alters the way we see both ourselves and others. It releases dopamine and serotonin – the neurotransmitters that enhance our mood and make us feel happy. Research shows that cultivating gratitude reduces cardiac symptoms, inflammation, neurodegeneration, depression and anxiety, while it increases hope, positivity, sleep and mood.

When we pay attention to what we are grateful for, we can reduce our worries and stress and invite more contentment into our lives.[1] Retraining our brain to focus on what we are grateful for also shifts our mindset from scarcity to abundance, and helps us to see the simple pleasures in life. We become less attached to material possessions when we start to notice the joy in the small things in life. Gratitude practices are especially powerful for transforming the negative loop in our heads into more positive thoughts and emotions. This builds our emotional resilience and helps us to find mental clarity.

PRACTICE: Keeping a gratitude journal

One simple way to become more grateful is to start a gratitude journal. Every night before you go to bed, write down three things that you are grateful for that day. If you find that you can easily write down more than three, write down as many as you like. Pick up your gratitude journal whenever you are having a difficult day to remind yourself of all you are grateful for. Notice how this practice shifts your thoughts and lifts your mood.

The power of witnessing the thoughts

We can change our thinking by cultivating *spacious awareness*. Put simply, this is a sense of distance between us and our thoughts. We become conscious of our thoughts by creating an observer or a witness state, where we come to see that we are not our thoughts, but the one who is watching our thoughts. Contemplative, meditative and mindfulness practices help us to drop into this spacious awareness.

Sitting in meditation to bear witness to our thoughts might be a daunting experience for some of us, particularly if we are experiencing distressing or anxious thoughts. If it feels overwhelming or unsafe to focus inwards in this way, we may need the guidance of a teacher or psychotherapist to support us in this exploration. For most of us with a busy mind, it is hard to drop straight into a seated meditation. That is why there is a scientific sequence in yoga to prepare the body and mind to sit in meditation. Firstly, movement through yoga poses (called *asana*) is recommended to prepare and open the body for sitting in stillness. Then breathing practices, or *pranayama*, are used to withdraw the senses, drawing us inwards to the present moment, where we can find a sense of calm. When the mind is calm, we can begin to concentrate on a particular meditation technique. We have already explored the first step of this sequence – moving wisely to create spaciousness and openness in the body, and in Chapter 5 we looked at functional breathing to prepare us to explore other breathing practices that can help to quieten the mind and support our meditation. We now turn to how the breath can bring us into the present moment.

The breath – bringing us into the present moment

So much of the disturbances in our mind are rooted in the past or in worries about the future. Our mind is so rarely in the here and now, even though this is the place where the mind can find a sense of peace and calm. The breath is a powerful tool to bring us into present moment awareness, to quieten the thoughts and to allow spacious awareness to reveal itself to us. Here are three practices, all involving the breath, which you may like to try to help calm your mind.

PRACTICE: Alternate nostril breathing for calming the mind

This is a breathing practice with a focus on calming and balancing the nervous system. It can be really helpful for slowing down the thoughts in preparation for meditation. Resume your comfortable seat with the spine tall. Extend the right hand into a fist and release the thumb, ring finger and little finger. Place the middle finger and the ring finger to rest on the third eye chakra at the point between the eyebrows. Rest the thumb on the right side of the bridge of the nose and the ring finger and little finger on the left side of the nose. When you are ready, take a full breath in through both nostrils, then close the right nostril with the thumb and exhale through the left nostril. Then inhale through the left nostril, close the nostril with the ring finger and/or the little finger and exhale through the right nostril. Inhale right nostril, close, exhale left. Inhale left nostril, close, exhale right. Please continue at your own pace, closing the eyes if you feel safe doing so. If the right arm gets tired, use the left hand to hold the right elbow to support the arm. If you can, continue this practice for two to three minutes.

When you are finished, allow the hands to relax to your lap and take a full breath in through both nostrils and a deep breath out. Notice how you feel and observe any effect of this practice on your mind. When you become used to the practice, you might like to add a breath retention or a breath hold – for example, you might inhale, hold the breath for a couple of seconds and then exhale. (Note: Please do not add a breath retention if you are pregnant or have any respiratory issues, including asthma.)

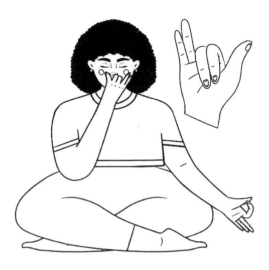

PRACTICE: Meditation to observe the thoughts

If you feel ready, we can try a short meditation to cultivate the witness state. Find your comfortable seat once more, either in a chair or on a cushion. Allow your posture to be comfortable, lengthen your spine and relax your shoulders. Start to notice your breath, letting the breath come and go naturally, without shaping the breath. Allow it to come in and out through the nose if possible.

Take a few moments, just noticing the natural rhythm of the breath. Notice if the breath is fast or slow. Now notice the mind. Is the mind quiet or racing with thoughts?

The rhythm of the breath is influenced by the mind. If the mind is racing, the breath might be quick and shallow. See if you can slow the breath down without holding it, just taking some nice, slow, smooth, even breaths. Invite the mind to notice the thoughts again, beginning to watch thoughts coming in through the mind. Sense or see the mind like a blank screen. Invite the thoughts to pass across the screen without getting involved, allowing them to come and go without judging them. Have the intention that all thoughts are welcome.

As your mind starts to become entangled or involved with the story of thought, just let the awareness return to the breath. Every time the mind drifts off with a thought, just anchor the mind back to the breath. If you feel comfortable, you might like to continue for a few more minutes, just witnessing the thoughts, allowing them to pass by and returning back to your breath. If you are happy to continue, now follow the inhale to the top of it, noticing the slight pause before the exhale happens. Without holding the breath, just notice the natural pauses between breaths. Likewise, at the end of the exhale, observe the slight pause before you take your next breath in. Take a few more rounds, noticing the pauses between the inhale and the exhale. Allow yourself to drop into the pauses between the breaths, resting in this spacious awareness.

After a few minutes, when you are ready, slowly start to come back to your breath. Begin to let the breath deepen. You may like to take a full breath in and a deep, sighing exhale. Coming back to your body, slowly begin to move your fingers and your toes. Gently come back to the space you are in and allow the practice to end. Afterwards, you may like to take a moment of self-reflection and consider the following questions:

- How did this practice feel for you?
- Could you notice the breath?
- Could you notice the thoughts?
- Could you allow the thoughts to pass by easily or was it hard to let go of them?
- Were you able to sense that you were not the thoughts but the watcher of the thoughts?

As always, if it was difficult for you to follow this practice, please be kind to yourself. Don't worry if you didn't feel any space between you and the thoughts. It can be more difficult when we have a lot on our mind. Take your time and be patient with yourself.

PRACTICE: *So Hum* mantra meditation

It is useful to give the mind a task in meditation. This keeps
the mind focused and stops it from drifting off with the
thoughts. In the last practice, we used the breath to anchor
the mind. But another method is to use a word or a sound
to help the mind to concentrate in meditation. This is *mantra*
repetition. There are many words or sounds that you can use.
In this example, I offer the Sanskrit mantra *So Hum*, which
means 'I am that'. This relates to our sense of oneness with
the universe.

Sit in a comfortable position to meditate. Become aware
of the breath and begin to quietly watch it. If you like, you
can close your eyes. Imagine as you breathe in that you
are breathing in from the navel or the solar plexus chakra
upwards to the throat chakra, and that as you breathe out
you are breathing from the throat down the navel chakra or
solar plexus. Sense a hollow tube between the navel and the
throat chakra. Allow the breath to travel up and down this
hollow tube. The inhale moves upwards; the exhale moves
downwards. It may feel as though the breath is lengthening
naturally. Continue for one to two minutes.

Now visualise the breath like a golden light moving up
and down the tube, and allow the awareness to move inside
the breath moving in the tube. Continue for one to two more

minutes. Now imagine the breath as a sound. The inhale is the sound *So* and the exhale is the sound *Hum*. When you inhale, mentally repeat *So* as the breath moves upwards. And when you exhale, mentally repeat *Hum* as the breath moves downwards. Please continue for a few minutes. Any time your mind wanders, just gently steer it back to the mantra *So Hum*, moving between the two energy centres at the navel and the throat. Continue for one to two minutes. Now, after the next exhale, we reverse the mantra. When you inhale the sound is *Ham*, and the exhale sound is *Sa*. This also means 'I am that'. Allow the awareness to stay on the mantra moving with the breath. Continue for another few minutes.

Then, when you are ready, slowly allow the awareness to come back to the breath. Begin to deepen the breath. Maybe take a full inhale through the nose and a deep exhale through the mouth. Very slowly, you can begin to open your eyes. The meditation has ended.

Consider the mind as a sum of parts

The inner landscapes of our minds are made up of a multitude of characters with different personalities playing out different roles. These parts comprise both the light and shadow that coexist in all of us. Our parts have developed over many years, creating patterns and habits that serve to protect, defend and guard us from pain. Often, some of our parts are working overtime to keep us from getting to know other parts of ourselves – the parts that we keep deeply hidden. The Irish poet and scholar John O'Donohue described the complexity and multiplicity of our mind in his book *Anam Cara*.

> At the deepest level of the human heart, there is no simple, singular self. Deep within there is a gallery of different selves. Each one of these figures expresses a different part of your nature. Sometimes they will come into contradiction and conflict with each other. If you only meet these contradictions on the surface level, this can start an inner feud that could haunt you all the days of your life.[2]

Becoming curious about the many different parts of ourselves helps us to see clearly and truthfully. Our parts are like our inner children, and just like real children, they thrive on attention and unconditional love. Some of them can act out or behave in challenging ways as a cry for help to have their needs met.

During his work in family therapy, Richard Schwartz began to notice that inside each of us is a system or family of parts that interact in dynamic relationship with each other, just like in a real family.[3] Schwartz developed an approach to psychotherapy called the Internal Family Systems (IFS) model. He suggested that our parts are influenced and shaped by our experiences in the world, and that they work together to serve our best intentions. He suggested that each part 'has a personality with different desires, different ages, different opinions, different talents and different resources'[4] – just like each member of a family.

No part is inherently bad, but some parts may have been forced into extreme roles to deal with our past pain, trauma and disappointments. They may be causing us to think and react in ways that are damaging to us or to those around us. Our thoughts and actions may be born out of fear or as a means of self-protection, and many of our parts are simply trying to safeguard us from a pain they think we can't handle.

Schwartz says that when we become a curious witness to our parts, we can have an internal dialogue with our inner beings. We can speak directly to them to discover more insight, guidance and wisdom. Profound transformation and healing can happen when we give each part the attention it needs. Many of our deep wounds come from our early experiences and the lack of support we may have had in the past, but as we become this curious witness, we are empowered to parent our own inner children. With awareness, we can speak with our parts, help them to see that we may no longer need protection, and give them permission to take a step back.

Can we love all parts of ourselves?

Accepting all of our parts fosters radical self-love and our sense of wholeness. When we acknowledge every part of us, each part feels accepted. We no longer fear our darker shadows, and we can welcome all parts with kindness and compassion. This helps our protectors to feel safe so that they can relax, allowing us to use their energy in a more useful way to propel us forward and not hold us back. We can unburden ourselves from the past, allowing ourselves to live and act fully in the present.

What is our true nature?

When all of our parts are in harmony and balance, we get a sense of our true nature. Hidden beneath the surface of our many layers and parts is a deep well of peaceful energy or spirit – the Self. There are many paths to get there, and regardless of what technique or tradition we follow – yoga, meditation, mindfulness, IFS, spirituality or creativity – this essence is available to each of us, waiting for us to drop into it. Some traditions say that we must master the ego (the external image that we have of ourselves that judges itself in comparison to others) – or get rid of the ego entirely – before we can access our Self. However, the ego is just another part of us that is acting from a place of protection. It has our best interests at heart. The ego wants us to survive. So instead of trying to rid ourselves of our ego, we can thank it for all the hard work it is doing. This compassion will shift the energy of the ego out of protection mode and resource it to be used for our greater good. When the ego is relaxed, we can access more Self energy, and then we can act from a place of wisdom and peace of mind.

PRACTICE: Tree pose

This is a balancing posture that can help us to bring the mind and the body together to find stillness. When we concentrate the mind in a balance, it helps us to quieten the thoughts. It is impossible to find balance when the mind is racing. Coming into our body in the present moment, we can feel calm and balanced within, and we can then carry these qualities into our life.

To begin, stand with your feet hip-width apart. If you want, you can position yourself close to a wall that you can use to help balance. Start to bring your awareness down to the feet. You might want to rock from your toes to your heels to feel more grounded in your feet. Then settle the feet onto the floor. Allow the weight to spread evenly through each foot, pressing the back of the big toe and of the little toe, and the heels to the earth. Activate the muscles of the left leg by pressing the toes and heel down, while gently lifting the inner arch of the left foot and engaging the kneecap. Feel the thigh muscle switch on.

As the left leg strengthens like the trunk of the tree, place the right heel against your left ankle. Allow the hands to come into prayer position at the heart. Focus your gaze on a point that is not moving on the floor or ahead of you, to help you balance. If you feel balanced here, you could move your left leg further up the standing right leg, perhaps above or below the knee. Press the sole of the left foot into the muscle of your right leg. If you like, you can raise your arms like the branches of a tree. Allow the breath to come in and out through your nose. Focus the mind on the breath to help you find stillness. Consider the feet to be the roots of the tree, the spine tall and strong like the trunk of a tree and the arms graceful like the branches. When you are ready, bring your arms back to prayer pose at the heart and lower the left leg. Now try the pose again, balancing on your right leg. You might find that one side is easier for you.

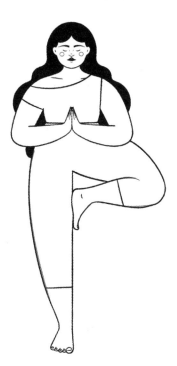

Can we drop into the wisdom of the heart?

As we find stillness and clarity of thought, we can begin to journey closer to the wisdom within our hearts. With a balanced nervous system, our protector parts relax and soften, enabling us to become open and receptive to the teachings of the heart. Here we can return to love and connection. These qualities nourish our personal growth and the seeds of transformation. Our beliefs, our attitudes, and even those relationships that we had given up on can shift and change for the better. To fully connect to the heart, we must release any remaining resistance or blocks. In the next chapter, we will try to drop out of the head and into the heart.

Pearls of wisdom

○ The mind can be our best friend or our worst enemy.

○ Our thoughts and worldview are influenced by our unconscious biases.

○ Shifting from a scarcity mindset to an abundance mindset has the power to change the world.

○ Gratitude helps us to nourish abundance and contentment.

○ Present moment awareness helps us to become more discerning about our thoughts and creates more safety in the mind and body.

○ Healing comes when we love and accept all parts of ourselves.

○ Our inner essence is the energy of peace and love.

CHAPTER SEVEN

Dropping into the Heart

"*These mountains you are carrying,
you were only meant to climb*"

NAJWA ZEBIAN

When my son, Woody, was eight years old, we moved from Ireland to Scotland, and he started a new primary school. My husband had accepted a job offer in Glasgow, and I believed it would be a great opportunity for him. We had moved around a lot as a family, but this was our first move since the kids had settled into school. My husband was hesitant about taking the job, because it meant taking the kids away from family and friends, but I reassured him the kids were young enough to adapt and that it would be fine.

Woody had been really happy at his old school and had lots of friends there since Junior Infants. On arriving the first morning at his new school, I watched him wander aimlessly around the yard on his own while all the other kids ran up to each other excitedly, congregating in different pockets of the playground with their different groups of friends before the bell rang. My heart was broken for him, but to justify uprooting him, I told myself that kids are resilient and that in time he would make lots of new friends.

He did indeed meet lovely friends in his new school, but his behaviour at home completely changed. He became very angry and aggressive towards me. In turn, I became frustrated and impatient with him because his behaviour triggered me. Our relationship became very challenging, and I took him to see a child psychologist, hoping she could help us to repair things. It appeared that Woody felt like his world was out of control, and he was angry that he had been made to move country and start in a new school. He blamed me for the move, and no longer felt he could trust me. His guard was up to protect himself.

After six months, I moved the kids back home to Ireland while my husband remained to complete his contract. It was a difficult decision to separate the family, but it felt like the best course of action to support our son. Woody thrived back in his familiar environment, surrounded by his friends. Meanwhile, both my husband and I had to navigate together the pressures of living apart. He felt I had encouraged him to move over and had now left him high and dry, and feeling guilty for all the upset in the family, I became defensive.

All of our life experiences leave deep impressions on us. Whether we are children or adults, we attempt to take care of our wounds by recruiting our protector parts. They wrap our hearts in thick layers of armour, attempting to stop us from experiencing more pain. Afraid to open, our heart becomes closed. Holding on to past hurts blocks us from opening up to new opportunities in our life. We need to feel the pain, acknowledge what it is here to teach us, and then release it. But so many of us hold on to our baggage. There is a certainty in our discomfort, because we don't know how it feels to be without it. As John O'Donohue observed: 'It is startling how desperately we hold on to what makes us miserable. Our own woundedness becomes a source of perverse pleasure and fixes our identity.'[1]

Releasing our blocks

By letting go of our emotional blocks – such as guilt, shame and past hurts – we can feel lighter, and our energy is replenished. We can use journaling or stream of consciousness writing to declutter our inner landscape. This helps us to pull our thoughts out of our head and onto the page. It frees up space in our mind and heart so that we use our energy for other things.

I first started this practice after reading Julia Cameron's book *The Artist's Way*, in which the author recommends a practice called 'Morning Pages'.[2] This practice involves writing three pages of stream of consciousness first thing in the morning. Carl Jung said that we are less defensive during the first 45 minutes of a new day, and that after about three-quarters of an hour of being awake our guard goes up. If we write our morning pages first thing in the morning, our ego is quieter, we are less influenced by the outside world, and our true feelings will be revealed. After practising the morning pages, our mind can feel rinsed and fresh, and it can be a nice time to meditate. We can feel lighter and ready for the day – and as we unblock, we may find that sense of dropping into our heart that I have referred to and become more connected to our creative energy.

PRACTICE: Write your way to an open heart

Begin your day by writing three handwritten pages of whatever comes into your mind first thing in the morning. Don't overanalyse it – just write down whatever comes into your mind onto the page. You might vent about things that are going on in your life. Over time, this process can be therapeutic and healing. You may notice the same thoughts and patterns are coming up for you, and it can help you to see what disturbances are getting in the way of your moving forward. The pages are completely private; you don't have to share them with anyone. Set your alarm about 30 minutes earlier each morning and go for it. You don't even have to leave the bed. Notice how things start to shift in your life.

Connecting to the heart chakra

Allowing our protector parts to feel safe gives them permission to soften their defences. Then we can begin the process of slowly and gently reopening the heart centre – physically, energetically and psychologically. When the heart is open, we can tap into the wisdom of the heart chakra and we can create space within us to receive what we desire in our life. If we hang on to the wounds and burdens of our past, by the time we reach midlife our heart will be compressed by a heavy armour of protection. We need to crack this armour open. To open our heart, a lifetime of fear must be overcome, but it is possible. The heart wants to soften and expand, and if we consciously set the intention to become more open, the heart will respond willingly.

Often, we confuse softness with weakness. But there is great strength in our softness. Walking through life with an open heart takes courage. The softness of the body is underappreciated. Stress and fear create tightness in the body, but relaxation can create softness. When we physically soften the front of the body, we can help to release blocks in two important energy centres that allow us to lead with an open and receptive heart. The abdomen is our core centre. From an energetic perspective, it is the location of the solar plexus chakra just below the ribcage. This is the seat of inner power. It relates to how we honour our Self. From here, we derive self-confidence and self-esteem. We find strength and courage to take action from our core. But we can also store worries and fears in this part of the body, which can contribute to tension and an inability to let go in this area.

At the middle of the chest, we have our heart chakra. This is our most powerful energetic centre and the most important organ in the body. It is our seat of love and compassion, and it is also the area where we hold grief and anger. It influences our ability to forgive ourselves and others. When we are overwhelmed and angry, it can manifest as tension in our chest, and it can feel like our heart is closing. When we are relaxed and content, our heart can feel softer, more open, and expansive. Softening the tension in the front body helps our inner armour to become more malleable.

PRACTICE: Softening the belly and opening the heart

Take a moment to sit or lie down comfortably. Place one hand on your belly and one hand on your heart. Begin to take some smooth, even breaths in and out through your nose. Feel the front body rise on the inhale and relax on the exhale. Notice any tightness in the front body. Become aware of any parts of the belly where you feel a sense of holding. Can you invite the belly to relax and soften a little more?

Now notice the chest. Can you sense any tension here? Could you invite the area around your heart to relax and open? Allow your awareness to rest on the heart centre. With every inhale, feel the heart opening and expanding, and with every exhale, allow the heart to let go of any tension. Sense that the inhale is nourishing and receiving. The exhale is a chance to let go. Begin to sense a light or a flame at the centre of the heart. As you breathe in, feel the light in the heart expanding, becoming bigger until it fills all the spaces of the heart. As you breathe out, allow the space around your heart to open even more. Fully drop into the light in your heart. Take a few more cycles of the breath. When you are ready, allow your awareness to come back to your body and notice how you feel.

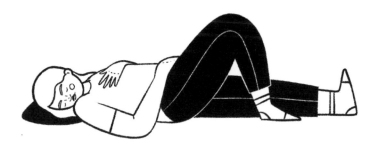

Healing our hearts

The energy that we put out in the world reflects the pain and suffering that is within ourselves. Critically, the relationship that we have with ourselves influences how we get along with others. If we are kind to ourselves, we will find it easier to be kind to others. If we are harsh on ourselves, we will be harsh on others. To heal the world, we must start by healing the relationship we have with ourselves. The inner work we do now allows us to consciously shift the qualities we radiate into the world. Coming into a more positive relationship with ourselves is the work of the heart. As we open our heart to ourselves, we can more easily open our heart to others. If we can accept all parts of ourselves without guilt or shame, we lower our defences and we can show up in the world in a more loving and receptive way.

This is heartfulness. The most important gift we can offer someone else is the energy of our heart – our love – and we are each full of love that needs to be channelled. We seek out relationships, looking for somewhere to put our love. It is our job to release the energy of love, not to store it or keep it hidden. Love is a light, a force for good, which we must offer out into the world.

When people experience a sense of being loved, they can evolve in positive ways. Experiencing love shifts everything. When we don't feel that we have love in our lives, we feel hurt and pain and we become bitter in order to protect ourselves, closing our heart. Self-awareness allows us to take more personal responsibility for how we are in the world. We are each a product of our life experiences and the relationships we have been involved in, the needs that we had fulfilled, and the needs that remain unmet. Co-authors Oprah Winfrey and Bruce Parry say that to understand human behaviour and the trajectory of our lives we need to stop focusing on the question, 'What's wrong with you?', and instead shift to exploring the experiences that have shaped each of us by asking, 'What happened to you?'[3]

Our emotional bonds and attachment

So much of our pain comes from our early emotional bonds or attachments and how secure we felt in our relationships with the main people in our lives. British psychoanalyst John Bowlby described attachment as 'the lasting psychological connectedness between human beings'.[4] Different attachment styles that we experience in early childhood influence our sense of safety and can have a long-lasting impact on how we relate to others throughout our life. In the 1950s, Bowlby and his colleague Mary Ainsworth differentiated between 'secure' and 'insecure' attachment. In adulthood, we may find ourselves somewhere on a spectrum between four main styles of attachment.

1. Secure: This is the most common style of attachment. Usually arising because our primary caregivers during our childhood were attuned, responsive and available to meet our needs. Securely attached in adulthood, we are comfortable trusting others and in giving and receiving love, and we can develop close connections with others.

2. Anxious: This usually develops when our caregivers in childhood have been unpredictable and inconsistent. They may have sometimes been available to us and sometimes unavailable. This can make us anxiously attached and, as adults, we might be insecure in our relationships with others. We can have a fear of abandonment, and we may need a lot of validation and reassurance from others to feel secure in our relationships.

3. Avoidant: In childhood, our caregivers may have been emotionally distant and unavailable. They may have been unresponsive to our needs. As adults, we can have an insecure attachment style, where we are afraid to trust and get close to others. We repeat the pattern of being emotionally unavailable and become overly independent. We may avoid intimacy and prevent people from getting close to us.

4. Disorganised: In childhood, we may have been afraid or suffered trauma at the hands of our caregiver. As adults, we are insecurely attached. We have a deep mistrust of people, and even though we deeply crave intimacy and affection, we are afraid to get close to people, so we avoid it at all costs.

Having a sense of our own attachment style can help us to understand our behaviours, our sense of boundaries, and why we relate to others in the way we do. What happens in one generation of a family influences the next. Exploring attachment styles is not about creating more blame in our families, it is about understanding how our early emotional bonds have impacted us. Maya Angelou once said: 'Do the best you can until you know better. Then when you know better, do better.' Our caregivers may have been doing the best they could with what they knew at the time. Shining a light of awareness on our own attachment style not only helps us to understand ourselves better, but can prevent us from repeating an inherited pattern in our own parenting style.

PRACTICE: Which attachment style resonates with you?

Take a moment to sit comfortably where you won't be disturbed. As you read the description of the attachment styles, notice which one seems to resonate with you. How do you feel when you think about this attachment style? Can you feel any sensations in your physical body? Ask yourself what feelings or emotions you can sense. Allow the feelings to arise without judgement. Just be an observer to how you feel. Take a moment if you would like to write anything down that comes to mind. When you are ready, take a deep breath in through your nose and a deep exhale through your mouth. Sense as though you are letting the feelings release with the breath. If it feels appropriate, you can offer forgiveness to yourself and to your caregivers.

We mask our pain with addictions

Attachment theory can help us to see patterns we have used to mask our pain or trauma. The pain might feel too great to experience, and we may turn to addictive behaviours or substances to bypass our feelings. Canadian physician Gabor Maté says that trauma, pain or diminished self-worth are at the root of most addictive behaviours.[5] Whether our drug of choice is sugar, cocaine, wine, shopping, overexercise, work or even spirituality, the addiction is used to stop us feeling a part of us that we have buried deep inside. Running away or masking our pain ultimately creates more suffering in our lives and in the lives of those who love us. Opening our heart to our pain, having a felt sense of it, acknowledging its existence and accepting that it is part of us starts the journey towards healing the pain. Then we can begin to see great wisdom in our pain. There are important lessons in our pain and suffering, and this teaching can help us to become who we are born to be in this world. As difficult as it can seem, we need to face the root cause of our pain to free ourselves from our addictions and reconnect with our hearts.

Letting go of harmful habits

I grew up at a time in Ireland when getting drunk was normalised and we were almost proud of our drinking culture. I had my first drink at 14 and continued to binge drink with the sole aim of getting drunk until my early thirties. After the dopamine hit of partying, a depressive crash that we commonly called 'the fear' would come – a hangover of anxiety, panic and dread. In my case, the fear would involve an emotional rollercoaster of insecurity, self-loathing and intense worry lasting three or four days.

On my hen night in Dublin, a girlfriend jokingly gave me a noose to symbolise how I would feel the next day after a drinking session. Deep within me, I knew that alcohol was not serving me in my life, but the concept of not drinking scared me. The only people

I knew who didn't drink where diagnosed 'alcoholics'. I didn't know how I would ever belong without alcohol, but I also really didn't want to experience the fear and self-loathing any longer. Experiencing two pregnancies back-to-back, I got to taste the sober life for 18 months, and for the first time in my life I found a deep sense of clarity and peace of mind. After my daughter Darcy was born, I decided that I didn't want to return to my old ways and wanted to continue my sobriety. But I felt self-conscious about my choice to be sober. It challenged other people's perceptions of me, made some people uncomfortable, and highlighted those friendships that were rooted in partying. As confronting as it was to consciously choose to live in a different way, the benefits were well worth it, and it has felt like one of the biggest gifts of self-care I have ever given myself. Crucially, it taught me that it is more important to be true to yourself than to keep self-sabotaging in order to fit in with the status quo.

The challenges of midlife can be compounded by old habits and patterns that are causing us harm. It can feel scary to go against the grain, particularly if those habits or addictions are more socially accepted, and it might seem easier to cling to old ways. But if you feel like something in your life is no longer serving you or that it is blocking you, it can be worth getting curious about how life might be if you could free yourself from this old way of being.

Facing our pain

As we begin to return to our self through our bodies, movement, energy work and meditation, a lot can come to surface. We might feel emotional after the practices and not understand why. Feelings like anger, rage, sadness or grief might emerge. This is a release. Many of us have been avoiding or suppressing long-held emotions. As we meet our body and our breath in the present moment, it can bring these feelings to the surface.

Even though it might feel scary, however, it is good to allow the feelings to come, acknowledging them and trying to find a safe release for them, either through movement, crying, shouting in a safe space, journaling or hitting a pillow. The emotions want to be witnessed and then released. When we acknowledge them and release them, we can move on from them, and this is progress. By releasing old pain, we free up space in our heart for new things in our life. As we journey forward, our intention is to integrate and carry the wisdom of our life experiences, but to leave the heavy load behind. It is not ours to carry. By letting go of the old, we can welcome in new and positive experiences that nourish us and feed our prefrontal cortex, balancing our nervous system and reducing our stress response. Finding more pleasure, joy and love in our lives is the elixir for our soul.

PRACTICE: Creating space for your heart's deepest desire

This is a simple breathing practice to let go of the old and welcome in the new. Start in a comfortable position lying on your back. You can bend the knees if you feel discomfort in your lower back. Bring your hands to your belly. Begin to breathe into the belly. Feel the belly rise on the inhale and fall on the exhale. Take a moment to set a *sankalpa*, which is an intention or your heart's deepest desire. Consider what qualities you want to invite into your life to help you achieve this desire and what you need to release that is blocking you from your desire. As you inhale, sense that you are welcoming in these qualities. As you exhale, feel the blocks leaving your system. Every time you exhale, sense that you are emptying out the old to create more space in your life for your desire. As you inhale, welcome in your deepest desire into your heart. Take about 10 to 15 cycles of the breath. When you are finished, take a moment to visualise what it would be like to have your heart's desire. Notice how it looks and feels to achieve your sankalpa or intention.

How do we let more love in?

Returning to love can heal and transform our pain and the voids that we feel. When we invite compassionate self-love into our own life, we can start to lessen our dependence on those substances or behaviours that are harming us. It takes courage to choose to heal your pain. It can feel overwhelming, and we don't always know how to start to remove what blocks us from living an authentic life. As we confront our pain, we soften our heart and come home to our inner power.

Affirmations are an empowering tool that we can use to start to shift our internal belief system. They are mantras that we repeat over and over until we start to believe them. At first, you might feel like an imposter saying something you don't believe, but very quickly, with repetition, the mantra will vibrate in your inner being and you will start to believe your own words. Siddhartha Gautama, the Buddha, is often quoted as saying that 'what we believe we become'. Whatever we put after 'I am' is what we become. Therefore, we need to choose our thoughts and words carefully, because our words carry energy and power. Repeating affirmations out loud can bring about great changes in our lives as we start to hear our words and begin to believe what we hear ourselves say.

PRACTICE: Create your own affirmations

Choose whatever qualities you want to invite into your life. With these in mind, write your own affirmations and repeat them until you believe them. Your affirmations may change over time as your needs change.

Here are some examples of affirmations that you may like to use as a starting point.

- ○ I am kind, compassionate and loving.
- ○ I am patient, tolerant and non-judgemental.
- ○ I am wise, worthy and beautiful.
- ○ I am able to maintain my boundaries.
- ○ I am able to trust myself to keep myself safe.

CASE STUDY: Eileen was in her forties with infant twins. She had relocated to Dublin for her husband's work, away from all her family and friends at home in Co. Clare. Every couple of weeks, her mother-in-law, Beatrice, would travel from Clare to visit them in Dublin. Beatrice would often go out shopping and enjoy eating out in Dublin. Although Eileen enjoyed the company and catching up on the news from home, she felt like she was running a bed and breakfast while minding two small kids. When Eileen came to do yoga therapy with me, she was angry that her mother-in-law did not offer to help with the children when she came to visit. However, Eileen never asked for help and tried to make it look like she was coping fine with the exhaustion of parenting young children. All the while, her resentment

towards Beatrice gathered momentum. Eileen
found it difficult to be around her, and after
every visit, she complained to her husband
about his mother. Eileen felt her own energy
was consumed with this grudge towards her
mother-in-law and she wanted to release it.
I invited Eileen to bring Beatrice into her
daily meditation, envisaging Beatrice receiving
everything that she had ever wanted in her
life. Over time, this meditation allowed
Eileen to shift the anger she had felt towards
Beatrice. She began to have more empathy and
understanding towards her mother-in-law. She
could see how Beatrice was lonely and really
enjoyed the visits to Eileen's home. Eileen
knew that her mother-in-law had experienced
a difficult life and perhaps didn't have the love
in her life that she needed. Eileen started to see
Beatrice through the lens of love and kindness.
Her grudge began to gradually weaken and
dissolve. Eileen knew that if she gave Beatrice
the love she needed, maybe she could show up
differently in the world. Instead of expecting
Beatrice to read her mind, Eileen began to
ask her to babysit now and again. As Eileen's
vibration changed, so did their relationship. It
is not always easy to visualise good things for
someone who has hurt you. It can take time
and practice. But it is worth the effort to try

to let go of the resentment we are holding towards them in order to remove the poison to ourselves and regain our own peace of mind.

Releasing grudges

If the mind is sending messages to the brain that we must protect ourselves, then our heart will close in response to the perceived threat. When we think about a person who has upset or annoyed us, we can feel ourselves triggered to close our heart at the very thought of that person. Holding on to grudges creates emotional blockages in our heart centre, and stress is a known contributor to cardiovascular disease. Even if we feel we are entitled to be angry, holding on to the emotions ultimately does not serve us and will only harm us in the long run. Do you know many angry people who are happy? The sense of righteousness we can feel about our anger is just our protector parts ensuring that we feel seen and validated for our grievance. Many people who have suffered great losses at the hands of others have discovered that forgiveness helps them to release their anger. They recognise that holding on to anger only hurts themselves. We can take inspiration from the power of the human spirit to forgive. Holding on to grudges does not serve us. We need to be able to soften and release. It takes conscious practice, but we can transform the energy of anger, hurt and pain.

PRACTICE: The wood chopper to release anger

This is a simple movement practice to release difficult emotions like anger. Stand with your feet a little wider than your hips and keep a little softness in your knees. Then interlace your hands as if you are holding an axe. As you take a deep breath in, lift the arms and hands over your head, and as you deeply exhale 'Ha' through the mouth, lower the arms towards the ground as if you were chopping wood with the axe. Have the intention with every exhale that you are allowing the emotions to come out with the breath.

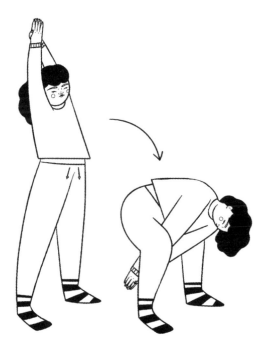

Repeat about 10 times. Be careful if you feel dizzy coming in and out of the pose. (Note: This practice may not be suitable for people with high or low blood pressure.)

Dropping our expectations

We all have expectations of how people in our lives should behave, and then we can feel let down when their actions don't live up to our expectations. Unspoken, this tension leads to bitterness and resentment. We can find a great sense of freedom when we release our hold on people and drop our expectations without compromising our boundaries. My father has a mantra to 'only lend whatever you can afford not to get back'. This applies to our energy, love, time, material possessions and money. He maintained that if you gave what you didn't expect back, you would not be disappointed. When we give with the unspoken expectation of getting something back, we set ourselves up for disappointment and we set others up for failure. If we want a thank you when we give, we might wait our whole lives for that appreciation. Meanwhile, we waste our energy holding on to that grudge.

As we have seen, boundaries are important in sustaining our energy. They are also necessary in managing our expectations of others. I truly believe in the goodness of others. But that does not mean that they will always act the same way we would. When we have healthy boundaries, we can keep our hearts open whilst keeping ourselves safe. Diminished self-love and self-worth lead to unhealthy boundaries. When we don't value ourselves, we radiate this energy out and we are more vulnerable to allowing people into our lives who manipulate and mistreat us. It is a vicious cycle, because the more we are mistreated, the more our sense of self is damaged, and it may be difficult to build it back up without support.

Breaking the cycle might require therapeutic support, because there can be times in our life when we need support to let go of old patterns. It is important to get that help when we need it, and professional support can have life-saving results. Unfortunately, it is not always possible to have access to a therapist. One of the consequences of the Covid-19 pandemic is that mental health services are overwhelmed with long waiting lists. Another barrier to access may be the cost of therapy.

If help is not available, in the interim it may be possible to do some inner work to consider what is at the root of our lack of self-worth. We can re-parent our inner child and offer ourselves what we now need most. Each of us is worthy of love. When we start to believe this, we can begin to value ourselves and treat ourselves with compassion and kindness. Becoming our own best friend can start us on the road to healing.

Cultivating empathy

When we practise empathy, we can see things from another person's perspective. By taking the time to consider how their life experiences have shaped them, we can come to see how their protector parts are influencing their current behaviours. Usually, they are acting out of fear. Seeing through the eyes of empathy facilitates healing in our relationships. In Harper Lee's *To Kill a Mockingbird*, Atticus says to Scout: 'You never really understand a person until you consider things from his point of view ... until you climb into his skin and walk around in it.'[6]

When we try to see life through another person's eyes, our perspective can shift and we can become less judgemental. We need to cultivate empathy for ourselves through self-compassion. We compare, criticise and judge others when we are insecure or feel threatened. By practising self-compassion, we can see that we are made of both shadow and light. We are not a finished product, but are constantly evolving and learning. When we accept that we don't know everything, we can find humility and grace. Then we can rest in the space of the heart where loving kindness resides. There we can remain open and receptive to the whispers of life.

Whenever we begin to question our 'right' and 'worthiness' to look after ourselves, we need reminding that we are upgrading ourselves so we can offer more love to the world. We need to honour the impact our healing can have on others. Our healing shifts the energy of the planet. When each one of us does the inner work to open up our hearts, we take responsibility for the impact that we can have in the outer world. Connecting to the energy of the heart, allowing love into our hearts and radiating love out, we can show up in the world in a way that creates positive change.

Pearls of wisdom

- To heal the world, we must start by healing the relationship we have with ourselves.
- As we open our heart to ourselves, we can more easily open our heart to others.
- It is our responsibility to release the energy of love.
- The challenges of midlife can be compounded by old habits and patterns that are causing us harm.
- When we understand ourselves better, we can stop ourselves from repeating inherited patterns.
- When we face the root cause of our pain, we can free ourselves and reconnect with our hearts.
- Pleasure, joy and love are food for our soul.
- Our healing impacts others and shifts the energy of the planet.

CHAPTER EIGHT

Meaningful Connections

"Connection is why we're here;
it is what gives purpose
and meaning to our lives."

BRENÉ BROWN

I met one of my best friends, Tonya, many years ago when we were both living in London. We had a lot in common – at the time both of us were married to professional soccer players who were away from home a lot, we both had young kids, and we both came from Ireland. Both of us were also trying to balance our role as mothers to young kids with changing our careers to pursue our passions. Tonya was moving from the world of insurance into interior design, and I was leaving academia to study yoga therapy. Away from the safety net of our respective families, we supported and helped each other to follow our dreams. We had each other's back if we needed help minding the kids while we took our training courses. We both became guinea pigs for each other when we were only starting out in our new careers. Tonya kindly allowed me to practise yoga on her and I benefitted from all her interior design advice.

Tonya was the one that took care of my son while I was in hospital giving birth to my daughter. She helped me pack up all our belongings when our time in London came to an end, and I was a support to her when she was going through a divorce. We forged a deep and meaningful friendship, and now, despite years of living in opposite parts of the world and seeing each other very infrequently, our connection remains the same. Whenever we do catch up over the phone or in person, my spirit is lifted and I feel energised. I believe that what allowed Tonya and me to connect so meaningfully is that we saw each other at some of our best moments and at some of our most difficult ones, and we never judged the other. We always remained kind, supportive and authentic with each other.

What does connection do to us?

As humans, we are hardwired for connection. Science tells us that relationships impact our health and well-being. Beth Frates, in her lifestyle medicine model described in *Paving the Path to Wellness*, cites social support as leading to a joyful heart.[1] In 'blue zones' – locations in which people are healthier and live longer – family and community are at the heart of the culture. Research shows that when we are connecting with someone, we mirror each other, with our heart rhythms, biochemistry and neural firings all come into sync.[2] Meaningful connections improve the health of our hearts and the health of those we connect with. And the more we connect, the more we jumpstart our wiring to connect. We shape the wiring in our brains through what we practise.

This is neuroplasticity. Shauna Shapiro, a clinical psychologist and mindfulness expert, writes: 'With every passing day we are literally training our minds and shaping our brains'.[3] Our daily interactions with one another are influencing our brain and our hearts. Shapiro says that we are sculpting and pruning neural pathways by whatever we focus our attention on or whatever we don't focus on, and that what we practise grows stronger. For example, if we are highly critical of people we meet, we are growing the neural pathway for judgement and criticism while pruning the pathway for being compassionate and non-judgemental. However, if we practise openness towards new people, we are influencing our willingness to allow for new relationships with others. By consciously paying attention to what qualities we are practising in our lives and in our interactions with others, we can choose which qualities we want more of, simply by consciously practising these qualities. This is how we shape our brain and break old patterns. Making small changes to how we show up in the world can have a big impact on the opportunities for connection in our lives.

The quality of our connections matters

I believe it is the *quality* of our connections that enhances our wholeness. And when it comes to the relationships in our lives, genuine connection matters more than the number of friends we have. In our era of social media friends and followers, it feels as though we often place more value on the quantity of friends someone has rather than the quality of those relationships. How meaningful our connections are will be influenced by how authentic we allow ourselves to be and how much of ourselves we share with others, allowing them to get to know us. For example, if we use social media to carefully curate what we allow others to see of our lives, often our accounts offer a fake or misleading representation of ourselves. A one-dimensional vision of our life can be disingenuous and might diminish our connections. If we are not ourselves around people, either in our real lives or online, we may miss out on making deeper connections.

When we change who we are to belong

Our desire to connect also means that we all have a deep yearning to belong to the pack. This need to belong has been useful for our evolution, and we have survived well living in communities. But it can also compromise our authenticity if we conform or change our beliefs and values to try to fit in.

I met my husband when he was already a well-known soccer player in the English Premier League and I was working in social research at Trinity College Dublin. In the early days of dating, he asked me to go out for dinner with two other professional footballers and their partners. I had never met any of these women before, but they were all well known, because there was a heightened media interest in the wives and girlfriends of soccer players at the time, and so I had seen lots of pictures of the women in magazines and newspapers. From what I had seen in the media, I assumed that they were concerned with beauty, fashion and high-end designer labels.

Knowing we were going for dinner with these glamourous women, I was intimidated and worried about what I was going to wear. My partner told me to just throw anything on, but instead I rushed out to the high street and bought a pair of ridiculously high shoes. Rather than focusing on the opportunity to enjoy meeting new people, I believed that in order to fit in that night I needed to change who I was and wear the type of shoes I believed the other women would expect to see me in. Despite having a stress fracture in my foot since my teenage years that prevents me from ever wearing high heels, I did my best attempt at glamming up and put on the highest shoes I had ever owned. Needless to say, I was very uncomfortable for the whole night, not only because my feet were incredibly sore, but because I was not being a true version of myself. This played a part in my ability to develop meaningful connections with the group I was with that night. I needed that lesson to teach me that I had to turn up as myself to find authentic relationships, and not dress up as someone else. As a quotation commonly attributed to Oscar Wilde says: 'Be yourself; everyone else is taken.'

What do we allow people to know about us?

We have many roles in life – we are partners, daughters, sisters, friends, mothers and grandmothers, work colleagues, managers and leaders. Often, we compartmentalise these parts of us, only showing certain parts to certain people. In the corporate work environment, we may hide our humanity in order to become business-people, and think it makes us look weak or vulnerable to show our family side. A few years ago, pre-pandemic, there was much fuss made of an expert delivering a BBC News report from his home office when his young children burst in unexpectedly looking for his attention. In the heat of the moment, the man chose to continue delivering his talk as professionally as he could, while his wife came in and frantically removed the children. This was a big deal at the time and the video went viral.[4]

Since then, the pandemic and the accompanying work-from-home revolution has helped us all to see the more holistic side of our colleagues, journalists, television presenters, teachers and businesspeople, as we have gleaned an insight into their home life through online video calls where kids, pets and partners carry on with their home life in the background. Our courage to leave our cameras on has offered a window into our home lives that has served to show our vulnerability and soften our hearts. As we see each other without the mask and corporate armour of the suit, we learn that we do not have to compartmentalise our humanness to be professional. In fact, how exciting and transformative would it be for our world to revolutionise our separatist approach to business and humanity by allowing our whole self to be seen – each dimension of us?

We deepen our connection and trust with others by sharing more of ourselves and giving others a full sense of who we are. It can actually enhance our personal and work relationships to see our commonalities, improving how we relate to others whom we might previously have considered very different from us. This creates a more unified and less divisive world and encourages more empathetic and heart-led leadership.

PRACTICE: The Johari Window

The Johari Window is a model we can use to build our self-awareness and gain an understanding of how others perceive us. It was created in 1955 by psychologists Joseph Luft and Harrington Ingham.[5] Using the model, we can explore what we allow people to know about us and what parts of us we keep hidden from others. It can help us to identity if there is a difference between how we see ourselves and how others see us, and we can discover what parts of ourselves we can share with others to build connection and trust. The Johari Window is divided into four panes of glass or quadrants: open area; hidden or façade; blind spot; unknown.

JOHARI WINDOW MODEL

	KNOWN TO SELF	NOT KNOWN TO SELF
KNOWN TO OTHERS	Open area	Blind spot
NOT KNOWN TO OTHERS	Hidden/façade	Unknown

1. **Open area:** This box represents the qualities, attributes, values and behaviours we know about ourselves and that others also know about us. This is the part of us that is an 'open book'.

2. **Hidden or façade:** This box represents what we know about ourselves but may keep hidden from others. It represents the parts of us that others only come to know if we choose to disclose it to them. We may choose not to share this part of ourselves out of fear that to disclose it would be harmful for how we are received or for our sense of belonging with others. For example, you may know you have a special gift or talent, but you choose not to share this with others.

3. **Blind spot:** This box represents what others know about us but we don't know about ourselves. It may include a part of ourselves that others see but that we are not aware of.

It can also include parts of us we imagine to be true, but which others do not agree are true. Others may see these qualities in us, but we do not see them in ourselves. We become aware of our blind spots through feedback from others.

4. Unknown: This box represents those things not known to us or to others. We may not be aware that we have certain skills, and others may not be aware of this information about us either. We are not aware of these things until we uncover them through self-discovery.

To illustrate clearly how the model works, here are some examples from my own life. In the *open area*, what people know about me — and what I also know about myself — is that I am a mother, a yoga therapist, a wife, and a lover of dogs, walks in nature, hot sunny weather and travel. In the *hidden or façade area* is the information I know about myself but which I haven't always felt safe to share with others — that I am a spiritual seeker and believe in a higher power. A *blind spot* of mine is that I can interrupt others when they are talking, and I am not aware when I am doing it even though it is obvious to others. This can be interpreted as rudeness and impatience, but it happens when I am excited to share my input and afraid I will forget what I want to say. In the *unknown* quadrant, I now know (but was previously unaware) that I sometimes experience anxiety in social situations. This was a part of me that I only discovered when social activity resumed following the early stages of the Covid-19 pandemic, and it is not something others would have known about me.

Take some time to complete the Johari Window for yourself. If you feel comfortable, ask friends and family for their feedback to help you become aware of any blind spots. As you journey through the rest of the chapters in this book, notice if you begin to self-discover any unknown areas of yourself that would fit the unknown quadrant in the Johari Window.

Taking off our masks

We all crave a sense of belonging, and throughout our lives we may have changed who we are or hidden parts of ourselves to try to find acceptance from others. Many of the relationships in our lives might be built on these false pretences we have created in our attempts to conform and belong. As we awaken in midlife, we can feel a shift in how we want to show up in the world and connect with others. We might not have the language to describe what is occurring, but it can feel like a heightened sense of urgency to make our lives useful.

To be impactful requires truthfulness and integrity, and to align with our authenticity and live from our hearts we must let go of our masks. This can feel like we are navigating risky territory, especially if we have a long history of changing ourselves to fit in. The people in our lives are only familiar with the version of us that we have allowed them to see, and this can therefore impact the dynamic of our relationships as we lean more into our truth.

As I embodied my authenticity, I felt a deep desire to cultivate more meaningful connections. The process of becoming more myself made me feel very vulnerable, and not all my usual friendship groups felt like a safe space. The dynamic of the group overwhelmed my sensitive nervous system and affected my energy, and it felt safer to connect with others on an individual basis. Meeting one to one, we could hold space for each other to go deeper in our conversations. However, navigating this period was unsettling and socially awkward. I turned down many invitations to meet up in groups, which created a lot of anxiety in me, because I was conflicted between doing what felt right for my well-being and not wanting to hurt old friends. Not everyone was ready or able to engage with me in this way, and my transition may have felt too intense or triggering for others. As a result, some friendships flourished while others shifted form.

This process can be lonely and painful. As our friendships evolve, we may need time to grieve. With time, we can come to accept and embrace these experiences as opportunities for learning and growth, recognising the great love that underpins all expressions of friendships, whether past or present, neglected or rekindled.

PRACTICE: What qualities do you want to cultivate in your relationships?

Take a notebook and pen. Sit comfortably and take a few deep breaths in and out through your nose. Ask yourself what qualities you want to invite into the relationships in your life. Allow whatever comes to mind to arise without judgement and write the qualities down. Now, as you look at this first list of qualities that you want to invite in, ask yourself what you need to let go of to have space in your relationships for more of what you want.

Then make a second list of what needs to be released. As the answers arise, try not to judge them; simply make a note of what you need to give up. Any time you need reminding about what qualities you are trying to cultivate in your relationships, return to these two lists and ask yourself which list you are practising in this given moment. Are you practising what you want to grow or are you in fact practising what you want to prune? If you find that you are practising what you want to release, be kind to yourself and start over again by consciously shifting your focus and attention to cultivating the qualities that you want to strengthen in your relationships.

Our romantic relationships

Culturally in the West, we place a huge amount of significance on our romantic relationships to satisfy all our needs. As women, we are often depicted as incomplete if we do not have a life partner, and often we look to these relationships to make us whole. This is a big responsibility to put on our partners, but we might find it is easier to look for someone else to 'fix us' rather than do the inner work ourselves. Traditionally, marriage was designed to support the survival of our species. Many marriages were not entered into for love, but to create political and economic alliances between families and to produce children. And it must be added that in many of these traditional marriages, partners were not always seen as equal.

Navigating midlife can be a revolutionary time for our intimate relationships. Gary Zukav, author of *The Seat of the Soul*, says that as we grow and become more authentic, we give our partners permission to be their full selves. This can bring more unity and harmony into our relationships. He says that in this sense, our relationships can become spiritual partnerships – a partnership between equals for the purpose of our spiritual growth.[6] The willingness of both partners to support each other's growth will influence our sense of togetherness. As we get to know ourselves better in midlife, we become more aware of the fissures in our relationships, and our inner healing might help heal and deepen the bond with our partner. For some of us, working on ourselves finally gives us the confidence to find our voice and fully express how we want to be in relationship with our life partners. Our inner wild woman might no longer be able to accept certain patterns that have not been serving us. And this might mean we find that our return to wholeness in midlife is better served by leaving a relationship.

Enhancing our connections through mindful sex

Sex is one important way of connecting with another human. By having sex, we can explore the flow of our own energy and we can exchange energy with our partner. Great sex can take us out of our heads and into our hearts. It releases endorphins and oxytocin, which allow us to feel pleasure and intimacy, lift our mood and deepen our bonds. However, our ability to give and receive pleasure through sex can be inhibited by negative past experiences or trauma, our relationship with our own body, our sense of embodiment, our stress levels, and how safe and comfortable we feel with our partner. Furthermore, as we experience hormonal fluctuations during midlife, our relationship with sex can change. Some women find that their libido drops and they lose interest in sex. Others report very painful sex due to the changes in the tissues of the vulva and vagina, which can lead to dryness and irritation or indeed prolapse. Hormone replacement therapy and vaginal lubricants can be useful to support us with these difficulties.

The biological changes that come at midlife might cause us to reflect on how we approach sex. The authors Diana Richardson and Janet McGeever suggest that conventional sex is not our only option, and that we might be better served by exploring tantric practices or a slow sex approach.[7] Tantra has its origins in an Eastern spiritual tradition dating back over 5,000 years. Visualisations, meditations and breathwork are used to explore sexual energy to build passion and intimacy either on your own or with a consenting partner. Slow sex is a mindfulness-based practice that encourages us to be fully present with the experience and to embrace a slower, more conscious approach to sex. Research shows that mindful sex can lead to greater sexual arousal and satisfaction and can decrease cortisol, the stress hormone that can prevent women from reaching orgasm.[8]

Growing up, many of us got our sex education from what we saw on mainstream television, Hollywood movies and pornography, and much of this content is centred on sex as a 'performance act', often with the emphasis on pleasing your partner. When we approach sex as something to be performed, it keeps us in our heads and blocks us from fully embodying and enjoying the sensations of pleasure. Adopting a more conscious approach to sex helps us to move away from what sex is 'supposed to' look like and from the whole performance factor. By coming into the present moment – being fully present in our bodies, getting curious about the sensations that we feel – we can explore what brings us pleasure and gain the confidence to share this with a supportive partner. Practices like tantra, slow sex or mindful sex focus on the present moment rather than on any expected outcome of sex, such as orgasm.

It is important to recognise that not all women will have enjoyed healthy and pleasurable sex lives before the changes in midlife. Exploring a mindfulness-based approach to sex, with the right therapeutic support, might offer us an opportunity to heal difficult wounds or trauma and find more sexual pleasure in midlife and beyond. We are often embarrassed and ashamed to talk about sexual issues, presuming everyone has great sex lives and that we are the odd one out. If you are reading this and sex has not been a source of pleasure in your life, please know that you are not alone.

When I was younger, I was in a difficult relationship that was not good for me. In an effort to control me and keep me in the relationship, my ex would insult my ability to have sex and repeatedly tell me that nobody else would want to have sex with me because I was so bad at it. I was very inexperienced, and the emotional abuse took a huge toll on my self-worth, my relationship with my own body and my sexual confidence. It took me years to find the strength and courage to leave the relationship and begin to heal. As part of my recovery from that experience, I sought help from a sex therapist to help me reconnect to my sexual energy and explore this part of me in a healthy and positive way. She introduced me to a mindfulness and embodied approach to sex, which helped me to find acceptance and love for my body. This augmented my ability to enjoy sex, as I dropped out of my head and into my body, and my propensity for pleasure was greatly enhanced.

Practising self-compassion can help us in many areas of our lives, including our sexual experiences. If we are critical of ourselves and our bodies, we may be worried about how we look to our partner. This creates anxiety and embarrassment around having sex, as we feel less desirable. The inner work we do now to offer ourselves more self-love and compassion can help us to feel more sexually confident. As we become more authentic and comfortable in our own skin, we can feel liberated to enjoy sex and feel more secure in expressing our needs and desires to our partner. The actress Jane Fonda found that sex got better as she got older. She said that she became less inhibited and knew what she liked, so much so that when she was in her seventies she said: 'I have never had such a fulfilling sex life.'[9] Yes, we might consider sex differently as we age, and it may not be as spontaneous as it once was given the demands on our time – we may even need to schedule it with our partners. Nevertheless, as we commit to becoming the most genuine and compassionate version of ourselves, it will lead to more pleasure and intimacy in our relationships.

Finding day-to-day opportunities for connection

Barbara Fredrickson, a professor in positive psychology, says that our connections give us vitality and that every interaction we have on this earth is an opportunity to connect. She says that meaningful connections can happen in the micro moments of everyday life.[10] When we smile at a baby we see in the shop, or thank the barista for our morning coffee, we have an opportunity to give and receive love in these micro moments. Having more of these micro moments of connection in our life can transform us – and the strangers we connect with – for the better.

To have more of these micro moments, we need to have access to others in our neighbourhoods whom we can connect with even briefly. Where we live can play a role in how we connect. The willingness and openness of our community to connect matters. Research shows that there is a relationship between the density of our neighbourhoods and our sense of feeling safe enough to connect with others. High-density environments impact our nervous system, activating our stress response, putting us on high alert, and obstructing our willingness to connect with others. This was my experience of living in central London, a great city with a special place in my heart, but so highly populated that in general people were not so comfortable having conversations with strangers. Coming from Ireland, the lack of micro moments of connection stood out. In my village in Ireland, it is commonplace to say hello to passing strangers, and every trip to the supermarket or waiting in line for a bus is a micro moment to connect. In London, by contrast, attempts to connect in such situations felt intrusive.

Our willingness to connect impacts the journey of others

Each of us is affecting the world right now, and no one is too small to make a difference. Every interaction we have is an opportunity to influence and strengthen the power of love in the world. When we seize the micro moments to connect with another, we send more love into the world. We can have a positive impact on a stranger's day. We don't always know what is going on in another's life, but our smile can lift their hearts and our own. Our brief interactions with one another may appear trivial and insignificant, but I believe that there are no accidents in the universe. Every interaction with another human is an opportunity for learning, healing and growth. Living from the heart, we can change how we think and speak to everyone we come across in our lives – including the person who bumps the line or the driver who cuts us off. We can consciously choose to react with kindness and not fuel stress and negativity in the world.

Create opportunities for connection

Many women have experienced isolation and disconnection during the pandemic. Their sense of belonging is fragmented, and their hearts are craving more connection in their localities. If this resonates with you, chances are that other women in your village, town or city feel it too. You may have heard a well-known saying advising you to 'be the change that you want to see in the world'. Often, we waste so much of our time complaining about what we would like to see in our communities without doing anything about it. But we can be the change-makers in our own neighbourhoods.

In my village, we don't have a lot of amenities that allow people to meet up in the dark winter months.

I wanted to learn to sew and knew that so many of the older women living nearby were talented at many crafts. The idea came upon me to set up a local craft community. Without allowing time for my insecurities to take over, I led with my heart and posted a message on the online community forum. Before I knew it, we had over 50 women coming together regularly to share different craft skills like sewing, knitting and baking with others who were keen to learn. More important than the new skills we learned were the intergenerational friendships and warm connections we made. In midlife, as we come home to ourselves and let go of our insecurities and fears, we can courageously sprinkle the light of connection amongst everyone we meet.

CASE STUDY: Kate was a stay-at-home mum in her late 40s. When she first came to me for yoga therapy, she was experiencing a lot of recent unexplained digestive issues. Her two sons, now in their early 20s, had both recently left home and moved overseas. Kate had a great relationship with her partner but they didn't spend much time together as he was busy running his own company. Both her extended family and oldest friends were living a couple of hours away. She had been close to other local school mums when her kids were younger, but now, with the boys grown up, these meet-ups were infrequent. Kate felt a big void in her life since her boys left home, and with a lack of social connections, she was very lonely. My instinct was that her digestive issues were related to her emotions. Nevertheless, I advised her to see a doctor and have some tests to make sure that there was nothing sinister behind her symptoms. The doctor could not find any underlying medical cause for her irritated gut, and after a few yoga therapy sessions together, I could see that Kate was otherwise fit, strong and healthy. As there was no reason why she couldn't participate in a group yoga class, I suggested that she join one of my gentle groups. I felt that Kate would benefit greatly from the social side of this group, as the women were very friendly and often met up outside of class. Kate agreed to come and within a few weeks she was going for coffees after class with the other women. She enjoyed their company and made plans for walks and dinners with them. She also joined a swimming club and her circle of friends expanded. From time to time I would check in with Kate after class to see how her gut issues were and she told me that she didn't seem to have symptoms anymore. It appeared that her health was benefitting from more social interactions and meaningful connections that were helping to balance her enteric nervous system.

PRACTICE: Seizing the micro moments for meaningful connection in your life

Consider how you can invite more opportunities for connection in your everyday life. Can you allow yourself to live from your heart as you move through the world and be a beacon of light to help people feel more connected? Take a moment to contemplate on what new opportunities you can take to find more connection with others. If you don't feel that current opportunities exist, ask yourself if you could be a change-maker and create some new methods for connection. If the thought of stepping into the role of a leader and creating new opportunities scares you, can you consider what is behind this fear? You might want to write your fears down to help you process them. Be kind to yourself and offer compassion to your fears. Then consider what you would do if you could release all of these fears that are holding you back.

Pearls of wisdom

- ○ Meaningful connections enhance our wholeness.
- ○ Being authentic and sharing who we are helps us to deepen our connections, develop more trust with others, and inspire others to step into their truth.

○ Midlife helps us to express the qualities we desire in relationships.

○ Our willingness to connect impacts the journey of others.

○ Every interaction we have is a chance to influence and strengthen the power of love in the world.

○ Embrace more micro moments for connection.

CHAPTER NINE

Trusting the Whispers

"*Difficulties come when you don't pay attention to life's whisper. Life always whispers to you first, but if you ignore the whisper, sooner or later you'll get a scream.*"

OPRAH WINFREY

was guided to move back from Scotland by my intuition. I could see that my son was struggling emotionally, but I also had an uneasy feeling in the pit of my stomach. I sensed that a darkness was descending. When I spoke to my husband about my wanting to return home with the kids, he asked me to think about staying a few more months and then we could all go home together. Normally, I would have taken his rational request into consideration. But in this instance, I couldn't ignore the feelings telling me to go. Within two weeks, I had packed up the house we were renting and had found my husband a small apartment in the city to rent, and the kids and I were on the ferry back to Ireland. We were settled back in our house in Wicklow three months before the Covid-19 pandemic hit. Had I ignored my intuition, we would have faced a lockdown in the UK with a ban on travel and no way to get back to see our family and friends. I truly believe that the sense of urgency I felt at that time was my inner guide nudging me to make sure that the children were settled back home before much of the world went into lockdown. To me, this was divine timing.

When we step out of our own way, we can become a clear channel to receive inner wisdom and connect with the flow of the universe. But when we spend too much time in our heads and not enough in our hearts, we block our receptivity. The mind creates much of our suffering, while the intuitive heart speaks only with love, offering us a deep well of wisdom and guidance for our greater good. As we quieten our mind and release emotional blockages, we can tap into the teachings of the heart. The guidance might be heard as the whisper of words or as felt sensations in the body. This is how instinct and intuition reveal themselves to us.

Fear disconnects; love connects

A consequence of fast-paced modern living is that we have become detached from so much that nurtures our connection to the wisdom of the heart. We spend more time in our heads and less in our bodies, and even less time connecting to our spirit, thereby fragmenting our wholeness. As we plug more and more into devices, we become more detached from the natural world and our place within it. Nature regulates our nervous system because it is our home, but pulling away from nature leaves us uprooted. A declining sense of community and an increasingly individualistic society heighten this feeling of displacement. Without our indigenous connection to the land and a sense of belonging within our villages and towns, we feel insecure.

Our nervous system responds to this lack of safety by allowing the survival parts of our brain to take over. In this process, we block ourselves from connecting to our heart centre. Fear and mistrust gather, taking us out of our heart and into our head. We need to find a way to feel safe again in our bodies. The heart speaks through the body, so if we are disconnected from our body, we will miss the messages of the heart, which are expressed through felt sensations in the body. Attuning to the intuitive wisdom of the heart requires that our sense of embodiment and interoception is not comprised. Remember that embodiment requires safety, so let's look at a few ways that we can enhance our sense of security.

Coming back to nature

Immersion in nature can help us regulate and feel safe again. The pandemic has been a collective trauma. To some degree, we all felt threatened and experienced a lack of safety and security. For some, the trauma was the infectious disease itself if they became ill and/or witnessed the death of loved ones. For others, the fear may have been the uncertainty, the restrictions imposed, and the loss of liberty we had previously taken for granted.

While our sense of safety was pulled from under us, we saw record numbers turning to nature for solace. Whether it was walking in nearby woods and forests, swimming in rivers, lakes and seas, practising yoga outside, people embraced the healing power of nature during lockdown. Many also felt the healing power of animals and got new pets. Consciously or unconsciously, many of us had an instinct that reassurance could come from returning to nature during this time of great fear. Our ancestors were deeply connected to the land and their natural surroundings, and that connection is still very much within us too.

In Japan, many people have officially recognised the restorative and therapeutic power of nature. *Shinrin-yoku* is the name given to the Japanese way of forest bathing, a therapeutic tool for health and relaxation.[1] Forest bathing is simply walking slowly and mindfully in the woods. It is now prescribed as a preventive medicine in Japan, and a growing number of doctors are certified in forest medicine. Yoshifumi Miyazaki, a Japanese forest therapy researcher, says: 'It is not just forests that have a beneficial effect on our well-being. Other natural stimuli, such as parks, flowers, bonsai and even pieces of wood have been shown to reduce stress, making these effects attainable to us all, even city-dwellers.'[2]

Being in nature is profoundly recalibrating for our nervous system. In the great outdoors, we find a sense of belonging that we may not have elsewhere. Nature brings us back into rhythm with ourselves and with divine intelligence. It is humbling to experience the energy of the sea, the flow of the river, the stability of the mountains and the grace of the forest. Here we can find a spiritual connection to a power higher than us. Nature is the great provider. It is a source of nourishment and replenishment. If we allow ourselves to spend time in the forest or the sea, we can find the safety and relaxation that we need to connect with our inner wisdom.

PRACTICE: Going barefoot in nature

Allowing time for our feet to touch the earth without our shoes and socks on can help us to feel grounded and connected to nature. This practice brings us closer to the sacredness of the planet and can leave us feeling calmer and more relaxed. When our feet make this connection with the earth, it stimulates the reflexology points on the feet, benefitting our entire body and boosting our immunity. Next time you have the opportunity, take a few minutes to stand or walk barefoot on the grass in a garden or park, or on the sand at the beach. Allow yourself to come into the present moment and feel the sensations in your feet as you walk slowly and mindfully, connecting to your breath and noticing how it feels to be surrounded by nature.

Soulful stillness

When our sympathetic nervous system is overloaded from sensory stimulation – such as too much time immersed in screens or living in urban built environments with bright lights and loud noises – sensory distraction makes it more difficult for us to naturally find mental clarity. It can be good to spend time in stillness to calm the mind and help us hear the whispers of the heart. It is in the stillness that we can reconnect with the inner landscape of our felt sensations. From this quiet space, we can connect to our intuition. To find stillness, we must slow down the pace of life and give ourselves time to just be fully present. We can create sacred pauses or rituals in our day that offer us the chance to become relaxed and that allow the golden nuggets of wisdom and inspiration to have the time and space to drop in.

A return to rituals

With life being so busy and chaotic, we need periodic reminders to slow down, pause and come back into the present moment, where our mind, body and spirit can integrate. In Dubai, I first heard the Muslim call to prayer and peace, the *adhan* or *azan*. This is a beautiful Arabic hymn played five times a day on loudspeakers to remind people to take time to pray. The adhan bathes the city in a wonderful sound at specific prayer times that are aligned with the movements of the sun.

During prayer time, people reconnect with their hearts, a higher power, the cosmos, nature and community. Even if we are not Muslim, we can develop our own individual daily rituals that act as reminders to take a sacred pause during the busyness of the day in order to come into the present moment and connect with intuitive wisdom. Anything can be a sacred moment when we use it for the intention of dropping into our hearts.

We can ritualise making our morning hot drink, taking our bath or shower, massaging body oil, lighting a candle or incense, saying a mantra, writing in a journal, taking a mindful walk, meditation, breathwork or prayer. We can get creative with whatever resonates with us to have peaceful moments throughout our day, offering us an opportunity to slow down and come back to our truth.

Nourishing playfulness

When our nervous system is in fight, flight or shutdown as a response to chronic stress or the result of trauma, we will be hypervigilant. Without feeling safe, our sense of embodiment is compromised, and so it may be near impossible for us to drop into our hearts and access the inner wisdom. Stephen Porges, the American neuroscientist mentioned earlier who developed the polyvagal theory, deepened our understanding of the vagus nerve, which as we saw is critical in activating our parasympathetic nervous system.[3] Porges says that the vagus nerve has two branches. If you think back to Chapter 3, you may recall that the first branch is the dorsal vagal root, which shuts down the body in the freeze response, causing us to become immobilised or to disassociate. The second branch is the ventral vagus root, which can have a more calming influence on the nervous system. Porges's theory says that playful arousal can move us more quickly from shutdown or disassociation towards sympathetic activation, from which we can then return more easily to a sense of safety. In other words, playfulness can help us to regulate our nervous system. To drop into our hearts, we must feel safe, and playfulness can bring us back to this feeling of safety. This science is encouraging us to become less serious and to invite more light-heartedness, good humour and fun into our lives. As we lighten up, we cultivate the conditions that help us tap into our intuition. So, play is not just for children; we need it too. The children in our lives are our greatest teachers. Let them inspire us and revive our playful side. Give ourselves permission to have more fun.

Expand your circle of love

Much of our personal growth is an inner experience, but there is safety, power and healing that happens when the energy of a group with a shared intention comes together. Connecting with others through a shared passion or a hobby – sea swimming, hiking, mountain running, crafting, yoga or painting – can offer us safety, community and emotional freedom to be ourselves. This helps us to come home to the heart. Since the pandemic, more and more people are coming together in safe spaces to experience releasing healing modalities such as breathwork, cacao ceremonies and sound healing. Women's circles are also becoming increasingly popular, using ceremony and ritual to offer women a safe space to express and heal themselves. Surrounding ourselves with like-minded people – talking and sharing in something we all enjoy together – can be a very transformative and heart-opening experience. Set your intention to notice what is happening in your own area and see what you are drawn towards.

Are we afraid to get to know ourselves?

For many of us, keeping a diary full of responsibilities and commitments is a tactic we use to avoid time alone with ourselves. We want all the noise so that we don't have to deal with ourselves. We are blocked by fear. Quietness brings us face to face with ourselves. In solitude, we see that our reality has been designed by us, and that we cannot blame anyone else for choices, decisions, actions or inactions that we have or have not taken. So we resist the stillness, making excuses that we are too busy. We tell ourselves we don't have time to *do nothing*. And many of us pass this busy habit on to our children, overscheduling them with structured activities and leaving very little downtime to just *be*. Our time commitments, rushing from one place to the next, create much of the tension and exhaustion in our lives. When we purposely divert ourselves from confronting our own inner world, we fill our days with any and all sorts of distractions and we miss out on a rich inner life.

PRACTICE: The power of daydreaming

When we allow ourselves time to do nothing or to get bored, we let our mind wander and we begin to daydream. This can be a time when we can receive fresh ideas, insight and inspiration. We may even find creative solutions to our problems. This practice sounds very simple, but can be surprisingly challenging when we are so used to distractions. It involves doing nothing for 10 whole minutes.

To begin, pick a time when you won't be disturbed. If you can, find a comfortable place to sit in a quiet space without the distraction of your phone, a book, the television or music. You can do the practice indoors or out in nature, or even alone on a train – wherever you prefer. Set a timer for 10 minutes and see how it feels to just sit with yourself. At first it can be a very frightening experience to just sit with ourselves. We may want to bolt and run away, scared of what we will discover about ourselves. If those feelings come up for you, acknowledge them and see if they settle. If the stillness becomes overwhelming, please end the practice at any time. Afterwards, you may like to take a moment of self-reflection and consider the following questions:

- How comfortable are you spending quiet time alone?
- How do you use distractions during the day to avoid being alone in stillness?
- How did it feel to sit with yourself in this practice?

Accepting our shadows

The current trend for positivity has put a lot of pressure on us to only feel good and show our light. A scroll through social media highlights toxic positivity, where only our best side is on show. In truth, the full human experience involves both light and dark. A refusal to witness and accept all parts of ourselves, especially our contradictions, suppresses our truth, which in turn creates more shame and guilt in our system. But concealing the dark feelings and emotions deep within us does not actually make them go away. They remain unexpressed. Denying our shadow is an unconscious form of self-harm, because over time these repressed feelings may manifest as illness and disease, screaming for our attention. By consciously diving inwards, we confront the muddy waters of our true emotions. Over time, accepting our true feelings helps us to clear the mud and strengthen our connection to our truth.

CASE STUDY: Claire was diagnosed with a very aggressive form of breast cancer in her mid-forties. As part of her treatment plan, she was to undergo a six-month programme of intensive chemotherapy, followed by a mastectomy and radiation. She was a very kind and altruistic soul who was always taking care of others and never putting herself first. As her friend, I joined her support team, and we made her self-care her priority. I began alternating weekly yoga therapy sessions and reiki to help her to rest and relax and manage the difficult side-effects of the chemo. With four gorgeous young children, Claire's will to be cancer-free was fierce, but after a few months of treatment she was struggling to accept the programme of chemotherapy. She said she felt like she was poisoning her body and she hated having to do it. But she was putting on a brave face for everyone else and didn't want to disappoint them. Working on her energetically, I could feel the fear gripping her body. I asked her to think about acknowledging her fears and helping to release them through journaling. Then with reiki and yoga nidra, we focused on releasing fear to make space to invite in a warm, golden light to heal her body. During her chemo sessions, she began to visualise the medicine as a golden healing syrup that was helping to cure her. Reframing her mindset about the chemo helped her to release her mental resistance and to find the strength to continue with the treatment. Shortly after this shift, she had a scan that showed that her tumour was shrinking. This gave her great encouragement that the chemo was a helpful ally working to heal her body. She has since finished all of her chemo, recovered well from a mastectomy and is in the final stage of her treatment, awaiting radiation.

Creating an inner garden of self-love

If we go to war with ourselves, we shut our intuition down. Our self-loathing stops us from trusting ourselves. So even though we may feel the sensations of the inner voice, we override and ignore the guidance. Without love for ourselves, we don't value and trust our instincts and we betray our hearts. But we are all worthy of love and we must give it to ourselves first. We can choose to love ourselves or to hate ourselves. If we don't have this fundamental sense of love and worthiness, we push away the path that is meant for us. Try to consciously choose to stop the negative self-talk and begin to accept yourself. Every time you hear yourself default to the voice of your inner critic, remind yourself to speak kindly and lovingly to yourself.

Acting on intuition is scary

It is one thing to create space to hear the voice of intuition, but it is quite another to act on it. Accepting our truth requires us to make difficult choices and to take action. Our fear of action can overwhelm us. We numb the pain of our self-betrayal by burying our truth deep down. Rather than being expressed, our truth is suppressed. What will be the long-term consequences of all this suppression? Perhaps we withdraw, unable to connect with others for fear they will know we are not being true to ourselves. Or perhaps we put up our defences, becoming easily angered and blaming others for our inability to take action. Whatever the result, the truth remains hidden inside.

We fear what others will think

Often our inaction is because we fear what others will think of us if we act according to our truth. As adults, we crave the same sense of belonging that children do with their peers. It is really hard to stand out and be different. We find certainty and security from being the same as others, even when going along with the herd is damaging us at the soul level. We each have our own unique destiny, but our fear of what others will think blocks us from aligning with our true calling. We navigate our journey through life pleasing others at the cost of what is truthful for us. Every time we say yes when we mean no, we are slowly breaking the connection to our inner guide and betraying our essential truth. We end up hurting ourselves when we do this. As we continue to turn away from this gentle guiding light, we feel lost. It can take a long time to find our way back out of the wilderness.

Intuition is our best friend

Our inner guide loves and cares for us like our truest friend. She loves us unconditionally, and so even though we ignore her whispers, she continues to offer us guidance and direction. When we ignore the whispers, intuition believes we haven't heard them and may turn the volume up. Disturbances in the body, mind and spirit may have to radiate louder to catch our attention and communicate a message to us. When we are unable or unwilling to interpret the message, our vitality can be

depleted, and in some cases this can have toxic consequences for our well-being.

How can we plug back into our guide?

When we are connected to our intuition, we are in
full alignment with our authentic path. Our journey is
smoother, our energy is conserved, and we are rooted
in a way that is true for us. So how can we tune into our
inner compass? No matter how disconnected we have
been, it is never too late to re-establish the connection.
The first step to becoming more intuitive is to forgive
ourselves for all the times we have heard the whispers
and the gentle nudges and have not paid them any
attention. Release all the self-blame, shame and guilt.
Then begin to accept that we are beings with a deep
well of internal wisdom.

When we believe that a sacred wisdom or intuitive
intelligence is available to us, we can begin to trust that
this source is acting for the greater good. We must create
space for the voice of intuition to speak to us. Slowing
down and allowing for stillness, quiet and alone time will
facilitate awareness of the inner voice. We can notice the
felt sensations in our bodies when we contemplate small,
day-to-day decisions. If we can listen to our gut instinct
on small, everyday decisions, we practise building the
muscle of trust to listen to intuition for larger decisions
in our lives. Intuition is like a muscle that we strengthen
over time with practice. If we establish belief and trust,
we can allow ourselves to receive the wisdom and act
from a place that is authentic to us.

Guidance from a higher power

By the time we reach midlife, we may have got used to life being difficult because we are not used to following our intuition, but it does not have to be this way. Of course, each of us will have our ups and downs and experience suffering, grief and loss. These experiences are part of life and out of our control, though they can offer us great insight and meaning. The path of authenticity is not about denying suffering; it is about leaning into our truth and the road that is meant for us. I believe that this road is divinely paved for us. The universe is pervaded with a great intelligence that is working for our greater good. This is the energy that infuses all of nature and sustains and connects each of us, and it is always sending us signs, encouraging us to follow our inner guidance. These can feel like coincidences or random events, but I believe it is often the work of divine intelligence or a higher power.

We collaborate with this great power when we trust our instincts, listen to our intuition and take courageous action to set the wheels in motion. Once we do our part, the universe becomes our co-creator and influences a cosmic turn of events that arises with a sense of ease and synchronicity. Likewise, when we are on a course that is not meant for us but keep pushing ahead with it, the universe sends us a roadblock to try to get us to stop. If we persist, the universe sends us more obstacles. So, if things feel like they are too much hard work and we are encountering roadblock after roadblock, it is often a good indication that we are on the wrong path.

I believe that if something is truly aligned with our soul, the path will seem more effortless.

Even if this is the case, however, when things are going smoothly we can then find ourselves thinking it is too good to be true, and self-doubt or imposter syndrome creeps in. We might even sabotage our great co-creation, believing it can't be real or that we don't deserve things to be so easy. When this happens, we can try to return inwards, finding safety and stillness to trust that everything is happening for our higher good. By doing this, we should find the courage to continue on the unique path that is destined for us.

How to ask for guidance

Despite our best efforts to work with intuition, we can still feel uncertain about what decisions to make in our life. I believe the universe can support and guide us with infinite wisdom, and that this divine support is always freely available to us. We just need to open our heart to accept it. People have used prayer for thousands of years to connect with this universal intelligence and ask for guidance. Some find solace and a sense of spirituality by spending time in nature. Others find connection in the quiet stillness of meditation. If you are unsure how to start, a simple tool to help you find your own relationship with this divine energy source is to ask a question and then journal the response. When we do this, the answers may reveal themselves in our stream of consciousness writing. Intuitive movement is another tool we can use to connect. Contemplate what you are looking for guidance on, and then begin to move intuitively. As we get out of our heads and into our bodies, the mind quietens and we stop overthinking. We drop into our hearts. We may discover that as we work the problems out of our body through movement, we have space to allow divine inspiration to drop in and reveal new creative solutions.

Divine guidance connects us to our purpose

Once we set the intention to work *with* rather than *against* divine intelligence, we can begin to marvel at how our lives unfold. Life flows more harmoniously, like an orchestra with higher wisdom as the great conductor, filling the world with sweet music. Opening up to divine guidance moves us closer to our truth and to uncovering our gifts and purpose on this planet. And as each one of us steps into our purpose, we nudge humanity forward.

PRACTICE: Reiki meditation to connect with our inner guides

We are truly in our power when we connect to universal life-force energy, or reiki. This is the force of love that supports all of creation. As we peel back the dense layers of past burdens, we create space to invite this divine energy in to support our healing. Here is a guided meditation with a focus on welcoming love and divine energy from the universe to fill our whole being. This meditation is based on the practice of reiki, a Japanese form of energy healing, and was taught to me by my Reiki Master, Liz Reilly.[4]

Find a comfortable seat on a chair or on a cushion. Cover yourself in a shawl or a blanket. If you feel safe to close your eyes, go ahead. Allow your spine and neck to lengthen and your shoulders to relax. You might like to rest the hands on the lap with the palms facing up, ready to receive. Take a moment to connect to your breath, letting the air flow in and out through the nose. Soften any part of the body that feels tense. Begin to notice the area just above the crown of your head. Visualise or feel a flower at the crown chakra. Invite the petals of the flower to open, revealing its centre. Move your awareness now to the third eye chakra, or the point between the eyebrows. See a flower here and invite all the petals to open. Now sense a flower with the petals open at the throat chakra at the centre of the throat. Move down to the heart chakra, the centre of the chest, feel a flower here, and invite all the petals to open. Now move to the solar plexus chakra, just below the ribcage, above the navel or belly button. Sense or feel a flower here and allow all the petals to gently open. Become aware of the sacral chakra at the centre of the pelvis. Visualise a flower here and feel the petals opening one by one, revealing a bud. Finally, notice the root chakra at the base of the spine at the tailbone. Sensing a flower here, invite each of the petals to open. Sense all seven flowers aligned along the spine together, each flower open and receptive, revealing a beautiful centre. Sense the spine like a tube or hollow channel connecting each flower. Each one represents a chakra or a vortex ready to receive.

Allow the awareness to come back to the top of the head. Sense or see a jug filled with golden light or golden nectar above the crown of the head. Allow the jug to pour light or liquid gold in through the opening at the crown of the head, allowing it to flow down through the channel to the third eye, then to the throat, pouring liquid gold into the heart, the solar plexus, the sacral chakra and all the way to the root chakra at the base of the spine. Feel the whole body filling up with the light or reiki energy from the universe. Allow this source energy to reach every space and cell in your being. Trust that this energy knows where to go. Allow it to reach the deepest parts of you that need healing. Know that this life-giving energy is infinite. You can invite this divine source in whenever you need it. It is always available to you. We are made of this energy. We just need to reconnect and welcome it in to replenish us. Take a few moments and bathe in this golden healing energy.

When you are ready, slowly start to invite each flower to close. Begin with the flower at the crown of the head, moving to the third eye, then the throat, the heart, the navel, the centre of the pelvis and down to the root at the base of the spine. Closing each flower helps to seal the energy or life force within us. Gently come back to your breath. Take a full breath in and a deep, releasing exhale. Notice how you feel now.

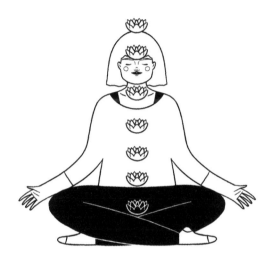

Pearls of wisdom

- Chronic fear disconnects us from our intuition; the energy of love reconnects us.
- Spending time in stillness and connecting with nature helps us hear the whispers of the heart.
- We can use rituals or sacred moments to drop into our hearts and connect with our intuition.

○ We can invite more light-heartedness, good humour and fun into our lives to nourish our connection to intuition.

○ Accepting all parts of ourselves – our light and our shadow – helps us to know our truth.

○ Nourishing self-love helps us to value and trust our instincts.

○ Ignoring our intuition leads to disturbances in our body, mind and spirit.

○ The universe is imbued with a great intelligence that is working for our greater good.

○ We can ask for guidance from the universe whenever we need it.

CHAPTER TEN

Awaken
to
Purpose

"Our deepest fear is not that we are inadequate. Our deepest fear is that we are powerful beyond measure. It is our light, not our darkness that most frightens us."

MARIANNE WILLIAMSON

I chose to take a hiatus in my career in academia to move to London to be with my partner and start a family. Becoming a mother in my mid-thirties was an awakening experience for me. Firstly, it cracked me open to experience the vastness of unconditional love a mother can have for all her children; and secondly, it showed me how much negative bias I had towards the idea of being a stay-at-home mother. Raising children is the most important role we have on this planet but also the most undervalued. In motherhood, I was afraid of losing my own identity. My ego was in overdrive trying to prove that I was more than *just* a mother and that I had something else to offer the world. At the time, my husband was living his dream, playing professional football in the English Premier League, and although I was happy for and inspired by him, I felt like the supporting act keeping things together at home.

Every day, I would take the babies to St Luke's Gardens in Chelsea, where I would so often see the same woman come into the park with her yoga mat. I was fascinated as I watched her go into her own little world, moving her body with the ease and grace of a dancer, as though there was nobody else around. And then when she finished her practice, she would glide through the park as though floating on air. I was envious of her lack of self-consciousness and wished to feel the lightness that she emanated. My heart spoke and told me to study and train to learn more about yoga. This then became my journey, to pursue my passion for yoga and nurture a gift I could offer others. Following my heart's desire has allowed me to live purposefully in a way that has brought great joy and meaning into my everyday routine.

Living from the heart

On this journey through midlife, we are finding our way to live from the heart. We all need a sense of safety, vitality and clarity so that we can drop into the heart to find peacefulness. When we ground ourselves in this heart-centred place, we can take action to be useful in this life. Being useful is what gives our life meaning. Research by Dan Buettner shows that meaning or purpose in life is one of the keys to longevity and well-being. He looked at five particular regions in the world, called the blue zones (referred to briefly in Chapter 8), where people tend to live longer. One commonality across the blue zones is that people here tend to engage in activities that cultivate meaning, purpose and creativity.¹ I recently visited Nicoya in Costa Rica, one of the blue zones. They have a slogan *plan de vida*, which they refer to as the reason for waking up in the morning, or a sense of purpose. Okinawa in Japan is another blue zone. Here, the culture recognises that we find joy in life through our purpose. The Japanese word for this is *ikigai*, with *iki* meaning life and *gai* translating as value or worth. It is our reason for being. In the yoga tradition, purpose is part of *dharma* – the path of finding clarity and guidance to carry out our unique purpose in this life. How can we awaken our purpose and find ways of expressing our wisdom to serve others in this lifetime?

The great divide

We are born with a light inside our hearts. If you have spent any time around young babies, you know this soulful radiance. Babies shine brightly because they are not yet socially conditioned to hide their light. As we grow and go to school, we are taught to conform and fit in. The education system is designed to turn out future employees for our global economy who will be highly productive and subordinate so that companies can make profits, often at the cost of human well-being. This process creates a hierarchy of worth, grading each of our personality traits, gifts, talents and abilities. It involves deciding what human gifts and talents are deemed important and worthy, while other natural abilities are deemed meaningless and frivolous. These constructs generate duality, divisions and power imbalances among us and cause a great many of us to dim our light so that we can hide or conform in a world that doesn't seem to value what we have to offer. Our wholeness becomes fragmented, and we see this manifest in our physical, mental, emotional and spiritual well-being and in our disconnection from our communities.

Tip If you have trouble accepting that you have unique gifts, it might be useful to visit the VIA Institute on Character, which has carried out scientific research exploring human goodness.[2] They have created a free survey to help you identify and understand the strengths and gifts you bring to the world. See: https:// www.viacharacter.org/surveys/takesurvey.

Our gifts and talents are divine

I believe that all of our unique gifts belong in us. They have been seeded within us from a higher power, with a purpose to help somebody else. When we fully embrace them and use them as a means of self-expression, we feel complete and more whole. Can we recognise that our gifts are the purest part of ourselves and that this is our sacred spark? We have each been tasked with a role in shifting the current landscape, and we do this by using our gifts: this is our greatest purpose. Great transformation and change are needed in how we live our lives for our healing and for the planet. The world needs leaders, change-makers and visionaries who challenge the status quo, push the boundaries and create new ways of being in the world. We step into these roles when we refuse to conform, choosing instead to use our divine gifts for their intended purpose.

CASE STUDY: Denise was a community outreach worker who was completing a PhD in psychology. She was in her mid-40s when she came to see me, to explore using movement to release trauma in her body from her experience as a Black woman growing up in an all-white neighbourhood. As a baby, Denise was adopted by a white family in rural Ireland. She had been the only Black girl in her school and her village for many years. All her life she had felt the impact of both unconscious bias and explicit racism. Her parents had loved her dearly and tried their best to support her, but they did not have the knowledge or lived experience to help her navigate and cope with the everyday discrimination. Denise was now the proud mother of a 20-year-old son, Oliver, and although Ireland had become a lot more diverse since Denise was young, she was concerned for Oliver as a Black man here. The surge of anti-migrant protests in her area was evidence that racial tensions were escalating in modern Ireland. Through her community work, Denise had got to know some of the women seeking asylum who were living in a local direct provision centre; these women

trusted Denise, as a fellow Black woman and
mother. They confided in her about their
experiences of racism since arriving in Ireland.
They had been threatened and lacked a felt
sense of safety. The women's stories resonated
with Denise's own. During our yoga therapy
sessions together, Denise said that although
she knew she couldn't change the world, she
wanted to do something positive for the
women in direct provision. She told me that
she had written to government representatives
but felt as though she was coming up against
a brick wall. The political system seemed too
large and overwhelming to make an impact.
She felt disheartened. I delved deep with
Denise about how she could use the wisdom
of her lived experience to support these
women. She felt that her mission was to show
them that they were seen and valued, and
she wanted them to feel supported by Irish
women in the local community. Denise used
her gift for community networking to bring
together a team of local holistic therapists who
volunteered to offer a series of self-care days
for the women in direct provision. The women
would gather at a serene venue to enjoy facials,
massage, reiki and nail treatments and to have
lunch with other local women who could
express their support for their fellow sisters.

Using the wisdom of her own painful experiences, Denise was able to create meaning and take purposeful action to positively impact the women in direct provision. She now sees this as her purpose and is driven by wanting to make the world a better place for her son and the next generations.

Remembering who we are

Purpose is not found outside of ourselves. It is a deep remembering of who we are. We live in purpose when we allow ourselves to be the fullest, most vibrant expression of ourselves. When we are brave enough not to become what we think others need us to be, we embody our true nature without fear or shame. Giving ourselves permission to express ourselves through our divine gifts is our greatest service to the world. This will look like a unique process for everyone, as there are many modes of expression. Our task is to come home to ourselves and remember why we are here, recovering our light and allowing it to expand and integrate into our whole being. This is the inner journey back to wholeness.

It is never too late

Many of us worry that we have left it too late to find our purpose. We may envy people who seem to have known their whole life what they are here to do. This can lead to us feeling like these other people are the special ones. But others can inspire us too. For example, when we see a great athlete, or a musician fully embracing their light, it touches our heart. It moves us so much because it is serving as a reminder that we have something beautiful and unique to offer too, if only we allow ourselves to put it out in the world.

Life is a marathon, not a sprint, and it is never too late to align with your purpose. Some of us are ready to express our gifts from a young age, while others need more time in the form of life lessons to shape and mould how we will express our gifts when the time is right. But our unique gifts have been inside us since childhood. We have simply forgotten, because of years of being conditioned into thinking we need to conform and hide what appears to have no value or worth in this society. As we peel back the layers and undo all the social conditioning, we realise that our divine spark has been within us all along, just waiting to be recollected. This is our homecoming.

Do you feel safe to be fully you?

Humans are hardwired to look for safety and a sense of acceptance from our tribe. Our survival has depended on this. If we don't feel safe, we live in fear, and we know what this does to our nervous system: we become hypervigilant and our fear shuts down our growth. We need safety and love to grow and become expansive. If purpose is expanding and expressing the fullest version of ourselves, then a lack of safety will inhibit us from our purpose. If we feel it is too dangerous to be the fullest expression of ourselves, we will contract, suppress and repress. What if the current landscape we find ourselves in – that is, the part of the world we live in, the values and norms of our culture, the family we are born into, or the community we live in – doesn't offer us support and safety to be our true selves? Then our strategy for survival might be to hide our authenticity in order to feel accepted by our community. When everyone else around us is conforming to the accepted norms and values, taking a different path can feel very uncertain. Nevertheless, growth requires that we push through our fear of uncertainty, and this takes immense courage.

Moving towards purpose can feel difficult

Awakening to the truth of what you are here to bring into the world can be a lonely process. It may involve disentangling from systems and relationships that don't support your purpose. For a time, it may feel like we are walking into the wilderness without anyone to guide the way. In a sense, this is what we *are* doing. If we have not grown up in a culture or a family that has supported purposeful living, we are trailblazers for ourselves and for those who come behind us. Essentially, we are illuminating the path so that others feel inspired and safe to walk it. This is the hero(ine)'s journey from the darkness into the light as we move from fear to finding freedom and liberation in becoming who we truly are.

The universe sends us what we need

In the Irish language, there is an old blessing *go n-éirí an bóthar leat*, which is often explained as 'may the road rise up to meet you'. Our job is to set foot on the road. With this action, we begin to align with our purpose. Then the universe will send us what we need on our journey. We can trust that the road will rise up to meet us. Paulo Coelho writes in *The Alchemist*: 'When you want something, all the universe conspires in helping you to achieve it.'[3] We can take comfort that even though this is an individual journey that each one of us can only do alone, we will not feel lonely for long. As we step into our purpose, like-minded souls will enter our lives to offer encouragement and support. Life will flow with a greater ease as we begin to swim with the current of the universal energy. This doesn't mean that we always feel confident in our abilities: we are human and we will have moments of self-doubt. We are engaged in a process of continually coming back to our practices to renew our self-worth in order to give us the confidence to push ourselves out of our comfort zone.

Purpose is heeding the call of our soul

Our purpose speaks to us through the deep call of our soul. Each of us has a yearning within us, and this longing is the song of our soul. It gently calls out to us, inviting us to remember why we are here. Ignoring the song of the soul, we are left wanting. We become restless because we have something within us that is left unexpressed. And even though initially it may feel safer to hide from our purpose, stifling the yearnings of our soul will affect our well-being, fragmenting us. Part of our healing journey back to wholeness is taking care of our soul. This is an intrinsic part of us that we must listen to, taking action to carry out the call of the soul.

The soul yearns for us to express our gifts through service

Talking about the call of your soul might sound very lofty and esoteric. Simply put, it is the expression of your gifts through grounded action that helps others. The world doesn't need saving – it needs our service. Consider the times in your life that have felt the most rewarding. Were they when you got new shoes, a new car, had the dream holiday? Certainly, each of these are enjoyable. But do the material things that we desire and chase ever provide the same fulfilment that we find when we act in service by helping another? Service brings us back to our humanity and gives our life meaning, and we can serve others by inspiring them when we show up with authenticity to express our divine gifts and talents.

Attachments block us from fulfilling our purpose

Our attachment to material goods and to the ability to acquire future wealth can block us from pursuing our purpose. The benefits of purposeful living have not been valued in our society, so we may have a lot of fear around how we can follow the yearnings of our soul and continue to pay our bills. Locked in a cycle of striving, we stay on the treadmill, trying to be more productive and to accumulate more. Because of the scarcity mentality that may have pervaded our culture, even when we have plenty we may live in constant fear that we will lose it. We therefore keep striving for financial comfort while pushing the call of the soul down deeper. Naively, we tell ourselves that we will finally follow our soul's desires when we have enough material wealth. Meanwhile, the years pass, we never feel like we have achieved enough to satisfy our perceived needs, and we suffer because we have repressed our true calling.

Inner peace does not come from accumulating more wealth. We nourish more joy in our lives when we lean into the call of our soul. However, we often fail to see that it is our current culture that is toxic and unsupportive for our whole being. We keep feeding this great machine, sacrificing our own well-being and, furthermore, passing these damaging expectations on to the next generation. This system can make purposeful living a privilege afforded only to those whose financial needs are met.

Life does not have to be this way, however. We do not have to feel so disconnected from the call of the soul. We can create a different life when we are not controlled by our fears and the old ways. Purposeful living and abundance do not have to be two separate roads. If we can awaken to the abundance that is already within us, we can radically shift our perspective to see that the universe gives us everything we need. We can receive prosperity by being generous with our gifts and by living our purpose. Leaning into a purpose-led life brings us more joy, and we come to see that we actually need a whole lot less materially. Our desires shift as our inner deficit is filled lovingly by meaning and service. Bravely placing the call of the soul at the centre of how we all live, we radically create an awakened life with comfort and contentment for everyone, not just for a privileged few. Any radical transition at the macro level begins individually with each one of us. As we wisely come into alignment with our divine purpose, we offer our service to help lift each other up.

Purpose can change through the life span

Our purpose can evolve and change as we grow and change. It is not static. Rather, it is dynamic, transforming with us as we develop and learn our purpose. For example, take the elite athlete who may find purpose in performing and serving others by entertaining and inspiring them with their abilities. Their gifts evolve as they age. The physical body can no longer endure the intensity of high performance, and there comes a time when they know they must retire.

But this does not mean they have nothing left to offer the world, even though the athlete may feel they no longer have a purpose after retirement. This feeling of a lack of purpose can cause them great pain, and often we see ex-sportspeople trying to numb the pain and loss of purpose with addictive behaviours. However, once they dive inwards, they may see that they have been presented with an opportunity to serve in a different way using the wisdom they have acquired from being a professional athlete. They might find meaning as a mentor or coach to those coming up after them. Or perhaps they can share their wisdom and insight as a motivational speaker, helping to teach others. Some might find that their gifts as a team player transfer from the world of sport into the business world, and they serve others by creating much-needed goods and services in the world without harming the planet.

The transitional period of midlife is often a time when we find our purpose evolving. If we have been parenting children, we will have dedicated much of our lives being in service to our family, and as our children become more independent, we may question how to find meaning in our lives. By contemplating how we can use our innate gifts with the benefit of the wisdom we have acquired at this stage of our life, we can find a new expression of service to others that will bring us joy and that feels rewarding.

PRACTICE: What is your purpose at this time in your life?

Take a moment to reflect on your divine purpose right now on this planet. You may want to have a notebook and a pen to write down the call of your soul. Sit somewhere quiet, where you will not be disturbed. Take a few slow, even breaths to allow yourself to drop inwards. If you are comfortable, close your eyes. Have the intention that this is a safe space for you to connect with the deepest well of wisdom that resides within you. Take a deep inhale and a full releasing exhale, letting go of any blocks you may be carrying. Begin to greet your soul, letting this part of you know that you are ready to hear divine guidance without fear, shame or judgement. Attuning to the call of your soul, begin to ask these questions with a sense of openness, noticing any whispers that you hear or felt sensations in your body:

○ What are my unique gifts?
○ How can I live more joyfully?
○ What am I here to do?
○ How can I serve?
○ What do I need to invite into my life to live a more purposeful life?
○ What do I need to release to live a more purposeful life?

Do you want to turn your purpose into your career?

Marrying our purpose with how we make a living can work really well, as it means that we are financially rewarded and gain meaning from what we spend most of our time doing. If you don't feel ready to leave the day job to pursue your calling, try to spend more of your free time expressing your gifts. Explore the possibility of charging for them and earning a little extra money. Dipping our toe in the water in this way helps us to see how it might be possible to make the transition full-time.

However, sometimes the added pressure of trying to make money doing something we love actually means we enjoy it less. If you have already decided that you don't want to pursue payment for your gifts, you will still reap the altruistic benefits. Living with more purpose allows even our mundane tasks to feel more tolerable, and we might find we bring more joy to our everyday jobs because we are happier in ourselves expressing our gifts in our free time. If you are unsure how to combine purpose and paying your bills, the pillars of the *ikigai* philosophy are a useful starting point to explore what might be possible.[4] This model helps us to identify where our gifts and talents intersect with a need in the world – then we can see opportunities where we might get paid for our service. Consider the following four questions to see if you can uncover new ways of earning money from living purposefully.

1. What do you love?

2. What are you good at?

3. What does the world need?

4. What can you get paid and rewarded for?

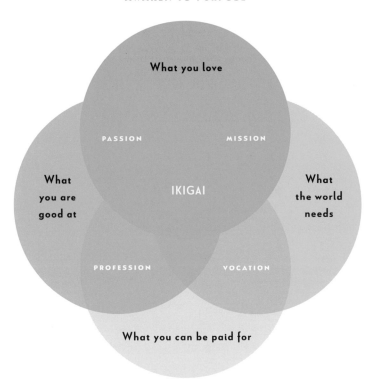

PRACTICE: The selfish hour

This is a practice to help you unearth and nurture your gifts
and talents. I call it 'the selfish hour', as it means dedicating
one hour a day to yourself to pursue your passions or what
brings you joy. If this feels like too much time to give yourself,
remember that there are many other hours in a day that you
can give to others. Use this time to cultivate your unique
gifts. If you are unsure what they are, get curious and try
new things that spark your interest. If you have an idea of

your purpose but have not yet felt ready to share your gifts, you can use this time to practise and build up the confidence to share your purpose with the world. If you are confident in your gifts and talents but don't feel you have time to use them, carving out the selfish hour will help you to find the discipline to set time to nurture your purpose. Use your imagination and get creative with how you use the selfish hour to enhance your life.

Purposeful living should not deplete you

Remember that purpose is sacred and divine. Sharing your gifts is your offering to the world. This beautiful act should nourish you at the same time as benefitting others. We are not supposed to be machines of productivity and profitability. Take time to slow down and cherish your gifts. Nourish yourself so that you can enjoy living with more purpose. Whether we are getting paid or volunteering, it is really important when we begin to serve that we maintain our boundaries. Serving is an energetic exchange, and we must be mindful of the impact on our own energy. When we are passionate about something and we see how it helps others, we want to offer more. This is great, but we need to manage our time and not overcommit ourselves. Very often, we undervalue our gifts and don't charge enough, or we give them away for free. This leads to resentment, because we haven't established a price that feels fair to us. Starting to value ourselves invites others to value us. Heeding our red flags and maintaining and refining our boundaries will help us to feel more resourced rather than drained and with nothing left to give.

In my case, holding space for others in yoga therapy and group classes requires me to be fully present. But to be able to show up in this way, time for my own practice is non-negotiable. Taking on too many bookings easily tips my scales off balance, and I quickly become angry and resentful if there is no time for my own practice. This is my red flag, indicating I need to find some free time by rearranging appointments or asking a teacher to cover a class. When I am mindful of my energy and I take care of myself, I show up better for my clients. With experience and hindsight, I have come to see that serving is about the quality of what I can offer rather than the quantity of work.

Fundamentally, coming back to our own boundaries and saying no when we need to, taking time out to recharge, and using our self-care practices to replenish and restore ourselves helps to keep us in check about what we need in order to support ourselves. It is also useful to question our traditional models of service. If we explore new, creative ways to offer our gifts, we might discover that we can expand our offering without burning ourselves out. Returning to our inner guide and attuning to the whispers of our heart will open us up to new possibilities and solutions that help us fulfil our purpose.

Pearls of wisdom

- Being useful is what gives our life meaning.
- Our unique wisdom and gifts have been seeded within us from a higher power, with the purpose of helping somebody else.
- Purpose is not found outside of ourselves. Rather, it is a deep remembering of who we are.
- Giving ourselves permission to express our divine gifts through grounded action is our greatest service to the world.
- The universe sends us what we need to step into our purpose.
- We can all create an awakened life by placing the call of the soul at the centre of how we all live.

CHAPTER ELEVEN

Nourishing Self-Expression

"The most regretful people on Earth are those who felt the call to creative work, who felt their own creative power restive and uprising, and gave it neither power nor time."

MARY OLIVER

Four years ago, I made a new year's resolution to myself that I would join a painting class. Art was my favourite subject at school, but apart from messing around with arts and crafts with my children, I hadn't done anything artistic since my schooldays. My soul was calling me back to creativity, and it felt as though there was a dormant energy within me that needed nurturing. So I signed up for a morning class in Enniskerry School of Art. Apart from the teacher, Louise, I was the youngest in the class. The rest of the students were retired.

I loved everything about the class – the art, the chats and laughter over endless cups of tea, and the teacher's warm encouragement that made me feel as though I could be as good as Van Gogh himself. The classes ignited my creative spark, and I began to flex my creativity muscle at home, painting and writing more and more. I believe in divine timing. As we align with the call of our soul in midlife, beautiful synchronicities occur that present opportunities for us to step into our power. From my simple new year's resolution, I found a great friend and collaborator in Louise. We went on to collaborate to create Art and Soul – a series of work-shops and retreats in Ireland and France, combining our passion for yoga and art and helping other women to connect with their creative spirit and enhance their well-being.

Creativity is the language of the soul

We answer the call of our soul through self-expression. Our sacred spark longs to be expressed, and it craves our time and attention. We nourish the soul through our many forms of expression. Creativity is the voice of our soul, but it can feel so exposing to step into our creative power, because we feel vulnerable baring our soul. This intrinsic aspect of ourselves may have been marginalised in our everyday life. Yet it is the soul that holds the key to inviting more joy, meaning and purpose into our lives. If we ignore our core essence, we not only hurt ourselves, but we deny the world our light. Reclaiming the soul in our everyday lives, we can become more present and joyful, and we can do this very simply by tapping into our creativity now, in midlife.

We are all born to create

The mistake many of us make is thinking that we are not creative. Traditionally, creativity has been thought of as something that is only gifted to the chosen few. However, creativity is part of the prana, reiki or energetic, vital life force that we each take in from the universe and that flows within us all. It is not something separate from us that we must go in search of. The divine intelligence of nature is the greatest creator. We are part of nature, and so inside of us we each have this creative potency. When we open up to our creativity, we allow the energy of a higher power to work through us: the universe is offering an endless stream of life-force energy, manifesting as creative inspiration searching for a human collaborator.

We are being called to use our creativity

As co-creators with the universe, we are born to birth our creative energy. Our ancestors were creators, inventors and makers. This energy is part of our growth and evolution, and it pushes us forward collectively. It is the force that helps us carry out what we came here to do – our purpose. Remember our divine gifts? They need to be expressed. By collaborating with universal creative energy, we find the inspiration and rhythm to dream our gifts into form. This is the great service we are called to offer the world, and it is not limited to just a few of us. We can *all* be infused with creative energy from a higher power. Julia Cameron, the author of *The*

Artist's Way, wrote: 'Creativity is God's gift to us. Using our creativity is our gift back to God.'[1]

By leaning into creativity, we reap intrinsic personal rewards, but we also manifest new offerings from which others can benefit. And this is so necessary right now, when we are each called to play our role in conceiving innovative solutions to the many problems in the world. Creativity is an internal superpower, but it is only by stepping up and becoming collaborators with the great creative spirit that we will rise up to become worthy guardians of this natural world.

Opening up to our creative potential

In many of us, this great power lies dormant, waiting for us to awaken to our creative spirit, and it rumbles like hot lava in a volcano before the eruption. Weaving our creative expression into our everyday life is part of our journey back to wholeness. The challenge is to change our perception that only a few are creative, and to know that if we remove our blocks, we can each become a channel for this playful energy. Osho, a spiritual teacher, said we must 'be like a hollow bamboo', ready to let this creative energy drop into us.[2] By clearing our blocks, we can be an open channel or a conduit attuned to the flow of the divine muse. In this sense, the creative process is a partnership, where we are co-creating with the universal source energy or spirit to birth new forms into the world.

Using our creativity is good for us

Remember Dan Buettner's research on longevity in the blue zones? He found that as well as purpose, another commonality across those areas where people tended to live the longest was their regular engagement in creative interests or hobbies they enjoyed.[3] Creativity can be medicinal, and it is now being recognised as an important pillar of well-being. Using this energy feels good, and when we lean into things that bring us joy, we move towards love rather than fear and enter a relaxed state. This activates our parasympathetic nervous system, which we know facilitates growth, repair and regeneration at the cellular level. This is all very good news for our physical well-being.

Engaging with our creativity is a meditative process. It offers us a chance to slow down and come into the present moment, giving us all the mental and emotional benefits of a mindfulness practice – shifting our perspective, enabling us to find more clarity, and enhancing our mood, which helps us to make better decisions. Using this energy, we can uncover creative solutions to complex problems. This has got the corporate world listening, with employers now seeking creativity as a skillset.[4]

Creativity flows with the current of life

From an energetic perspective, untapped creativity can cause blockages in our system. This might manifest as an unexplained sense of frustration, restlessness, anger and discontentment. Chronically repressing this energy might make us ill. Without an outlet for our expression, it may even lead us into a sense of depression. When we use our creativity, we can feel truly alive. This energy will bring us into a flow state or a sense that we are 'in the zone'. This is a powerful state of clarity that can feel blissful or ecstatic, because we lose all sense of self-doubt and worry as we become completely absorbed in what we are doing. In these precious moments, time seems to stand still, because we are so focused on what we are doing. There is a sense of effortlessness and a harmony of flow.

What blocks us from creative self-expression?

Through the global scarcity mindset, we have been pitted against each other in all aspects of our lives, and creativity is no exception. This mindset fuels the idea that one person's creative talent or success means that there is less to go around for the rest of us. What if we could trust that there is an abundance of creative energy in the universe? When we realise that there is enough to go around for everyone, we can accept that to be human is to be innately creative. We come to know then that we are not in competition with anyone else and that we are all artists with different gifts and talents that take many forms. Creative energy runs through our whole being, waiting for the chance to be expressed.

Can we allow ourselves more joy?

If we look at the values in our society, it seems that we have come to believe that life should be hard. We have a strong work ethic at a cost to our health. Stress is normalised and burnout is common, perhaps especially in midlife. We are time poor and our relationships suffer, and we try to find our worth and value in how busy and overworked we are. We hurry our kids and overburden them, socialising them into this toxic culture. We not only perceive that life is hard, but we believe that there is no other way to live.

When it comes to nourishing our soul through creativity and joy, we are so disconnected from accepting joy as part of life that we don't accept that we deserve it. It can feel greedy and self-indulgent. But joy is our birthright. It is very simple: our current model of living is out of alignment with what we are here to experience. We have been culturally programmed to live in a way that encourages more pain than pleasure. It is time to invite more joy into our lives by living a more creative life. *Simply flexing our creative muscle for the sake of joy is a crucial pillar for our well-being and has far-reaching benefits for the greater good.*

Can we trust that we are co-creators?

When we begin to trust in something greater than us, it can remove the responsibility of the creative outcome from us personally. If we are channelling inspiration from a higher source, then the burden of whether it is good or bad is irrelevant to us, and we are free from external judgement. The creative process is a metaphor for life. We do not know the outcome. The story unfolds as we journey through the process, and we just need to trust and surrender to the process. By turning the tap on, we allow the stream of creativity to flow.

Starting to value creativity in our lives

Despite the massive benefits we reap from creativity, we have left very little time for it in our busy, modern lives. A slower pace of life and the lack of mass production allowed our ancestors to express their creativity through everyday activities such as baking, cooking, foraging, gardening, dressmaking and woodwork – to name just a few. Many of us have lost that creative expression in the pace of our everyday lives, and we no longer value the process of creativity.

Even if we do agree that we have something to express creatively, we have been culturally conditioned to channel this energy, if possible, into earning money, recognition or critical acclaim. While there is nothing wrong with earning money from our talents, and it can be good to do so (see Chapter 10), sometimes the emphasis is on the outcome and not on what the creative process itself has to offer. We have not been taught to express our creative side for the joy and pleasure it can bring us (which translates into significant health benefits) or for how it can serve others. And unless we are a professional creative (that is, we get paid to be creative for a living), we typically accept that only two cohorts should indulge in creativity for the sake of it: children and older people. It is accepted that retired people can afford to be self-indulgent with creative pursuits because they have the luxury of free time, and creative pursuits are a natural part of a child's life and play.

But through our children, we may sometimes aspire to fulfil our own unmet creativity needs. As parents, many of us choose activities for our kids that we wish we had done, and in doing so we may put them under pressure to answer the yearnings of our own soul rather than of theirs. They cannot fulfil our soul's passions, however: only we can do that for ourselves through our own self-expression.

Perfection is the enemy of action

Because we may have valued only the outcomes rather than the process, we may fear that our creative efforts will not be good enough. Afraid that we are not wise enough, qualified enough or prepared enough, most of us never begin. Our desire to be perfect prevents us from trying.

Wabi-sabi is a philosophy in Japan that suggests that life is more beautiful the less perfect it is and that there is great beauty in our imperfections.[5] If we adapt this principal to our creative self-expression, we can take solace knowing that 'perfect' does not exist. Creativity requires a radical state of self-acceptance. If we can accept and love all parts of ourselves, including our imperfections, then we can give ourselves permission in midlife to explore our creative expression.

Dropping into the qualities of the heart, we can see ourselves with kindness and compassion. Accepting our humanity and the fact that sometimes we make mistakes, can we be brave enough to try new things even if we fail? Can we see mistakes as opportunities for learning, growth and evolution? This takes courage, vulnerability and continued work until we have healed our deep wounds.

We find excuses to not try

Our excuses are often only our fears in disguise. Lack of time is a great reason we give not to create, especially in midlife when we may have many responsibilities. But we may be surprised if we check our screen time on our phone to see how much wasted time could have been spent creating. Glennon Doyle, author and mother, said she found time in her day to write by giving up evening TV, going to bed and getting up to write in the early morning hours.[6] Money is another excuse that is often used, even though it does not always need to be an obstacle. Many of our creative passions do not need to cost anything.

Using our parenting responsibilities as an excuse doesn't hold up either, even at this busy stage of midlife. If you are a parent, you know it is nigh on impossible to lock yourself away in a studio and create to your heart's content – we often have to grab the snippets of time that are available between work, domestic responsibilities and parenting. But by expressing our creativity in this way, we can still be a role model to our children. A lot of soulful, joyful and creative things can be done while also being present with our children. Emma Donoghue, novelist and screenwriter, told of how she wrote her novel *Room*[7] while her children ran around the house. My good friend Louise is an artist and mother to eight children. She works on her paintings in an open studio she created in a small passageway between her kitchen and sitting room, right in the thick of the family. When we make creativity visible to our children, we inspire them to live an authentic life that includes varied ways in which they can express themselves.

Self-expression requires vulnerability

Allowing ourselves to create is an act of bravery as we become vulnerable to other people's opinions. However, what others think of us is actually none of our business. When we begin to try new things, it may make people in our lives uncomfortable. Human nature does not like uncertainty and change, and we like to keep people in certain boxes. This makes us feel safer. And if we find that we too are uncomfortable when people in our lives start doing new things, it may be a reflection of some deep yearnings within ourselves. Emotions like jealousy or envy can show up to teach us about what we want more of in our own life. They challenge us to think about how we are living, and we can use these emotions wisely, allowing them to reveal to us how we feel called to express ourselves.

CASE STUDY: Wanda was 47. Her whole life, she had found it difficult to express herself and often felt angry inside. Physically, she held a lot of tension in her chest, neck, shoulders and jaw. She had always wanted to pursue a career as an artist, but she was afraid she wouldn't be good enough. Her mother was an artist and had been highly critical of her as child. Even now in her middle years, Wanda was afraid her mother would judge her harshly. While running an art and yoga workshop, I had seen some of Wanda's work. She was extremely talented, but moreover I could see the immense pleasure she got from painting. Practising art, she lost herself in the moment and it became meditative and relaxing for her. I also noticed that Wanda was very hard on herself and very disparaging of her work. During the workshop, I invited the group to sing a mantra together. Mantras are ancient sacred sounds that can be used for healing our energy centres and raising our vibrations. I encouraged Wanda to practise a mantra daily with the intention of clearing her throat chakra in order to gain the confidence to use her voice to express herself and her inner artist.

PRACTICE: The bija mantras

The *bija* mantras, also known as *seed* mantras, are transformative sounds associated with the seven chakras or energy centres in the body. To help to clear the chakras, repeat all seven sounds out loud. Sit comfortably in a meditative position. Allow your awareness to move inwards. Focus your attention onto the area of the body related to each chakra as you chant the sound.

1. **Base chakra:** Place the awareness on the base of the spine and chant LAM.

2. **Sacral chakra:** Place the awareness on the pelvis and chant VAM.

3. **Solar plexus chakra:** Place the awareness on the navel centre and chant RAM.

4. **Heart chakra:** Place the awareness on the heart and chant YAM.

5. **Throat chakra:** Place the awareness on the throat and chant HAM.

6. **Third eye chakra:** Place the awareness on the point between the eyebrows and chant OM.

7. **Crown chakra:** Place your awareness on the crown of the head and chant a silent OM.

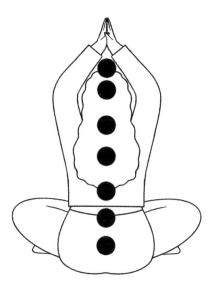

Resisting the temptation of distractions

Can you remember a time back in school when you had to study or meet a deadline, but you found yourself wanting to do anything other than the task at hand? All of a sudden, tidying up, doing the laundry – or any other mundane task – felt better than actually sitting down and doing the work. The same is true with creativity in midlife. Rather than face head-on what we want to explore, we procrastinate and find things that divert our focus, because we fear failure and disappointment. We tell ourselves we will get started when the house is clean, the laundry is done, the groceries are bought. And we end up never getting started. Can you give yourself an hour to connect with the creative spirit before you do the endless list of chores?

How to invite more creativity in

If we feel we are not creative, we are simply disconnected from this part of ourselves. While we have been passively consuming the creations of others, it is possible that we have closed ourselves off to our own creative capacities and the spirit of divine inspiration. Reminding ourselves of how naturally we embraced creative expression as children and adolescents can help us, in midlife, to believe that we once had this connection. And it is possible to start to rebuild it.

Consider what creative ways you used in order to express yourself when you were younger. It might have been inventing, doing science experiments, making up plays, dressing up, designing and making clothes, singing, dancing, making pretend radio or TV shows, art, sport, building forts, craft-making, cooking, gardening – you may have numerous passions on your list. Our interests as children are usually a good guide as to what methods of self-expression might make our soul sing now in midlife. As a child, I loved dancing, writing stories and art. Now I express my creative energy through yoga, intuitive movement, painting and writing. Once we remember what brings us joy, it is important that we find ways to make these things part of our daily life. The more we cultivate our joyful experiences, the less room there is for our fears to block our inner artist.

Slowing down to create space for inspiration

Creativity is not productivity. It requires time to do nothing, in quietness and stillness – time to daydream and doodle so that there is open space to let inspiration come in. It can arrive without warning and can feel unpredictable, but also playful and fun. We must be ready to move with the rhythm of the creative spirit. It might arrive like a giant surge or like gentle ripples, and we must be ready to move in right rhythm to receive its guidance.

We also need time to rest after dancing with the flow of creativity – to refresh, recharge and prepare ourselves for the next surge of inspiration whenever it arrives. Of course, some days will feel more inspiring than others. This is normal and natural. It is good to take each day as it comes, allowing the creative experience to unfold naturally and without force, knowing that tomorrow brings another day for us to show up with the intention of staying open to receiving the gift of creativity, to shine our light and express our gifts.

PRACTICE: Finding your own ritual to prepare to open up to creativity

It can be useful to have routines or rituals that you use to make space for the creative force to come through you. Here are some examples of what I like to do to open up space to work creatively.

Movement: Spend a few minutes moving your body intuitively in ways that feel good to help you let go of tension and tightness and create room and space in your physical body to work creatively.

Breathing: We can use the breath to help us let go of old ways in order to make space for new ideas and inspiration. Take about five deep breaths in and out, with an emphasis on the exhale as a chance to release and let go, while the inhale is an opportunity to take in the new. With every cycle of the breath, we feel lighter as we make space to welcome in fresh ideas.

Create a sacred space: Cleanse and purify the energy of your space to welcome in creativity by lighting a candle or incense, or by using a smudging ritual with wood sticks like sage or palo santo.

Set an intention: An intention is something that we want to invite into our life. Perhaps the intention is simply that we are opening ourselves to divine inspiration and creativity. Whatever our intention, we can say it out loud or write it down. After we set the intention, we can just release all attachment to what comes next and allow things to unfold.

Meditation: You might like to meditate for a few minutes, dropping into your heart to find peaceful stillness to attune to creative inspiration.

Try to have fun with creative energy

It takes courage and vulnerability to tap into our creativity, especially in midlife, if it is some time since we have tried it, but it is also extremely worthwhile and pleasurable. Just a few minutes a day exploring our creativity helps us to reconnect with this part of ourselves. Over time, we might enjoy the process so much that a few minutes becomes a few hours. We might find that we sacrifice Netflix or scrolling through Instagram, and before we know it, we might have tipped the scales and find ourselves spending much more of our free time connecting with our creative spirit. As we come back to our creativity, we can find that our perspective shifts. We access new parts of our consciousness and change old habits and patterns. We invite new things into our lives and find it easier to let go of things that were no longer serving us.

Pearls of wisdom

- ○ We answer the call of our soul through the energy of creativity.
- ○ We are all born to co-create with the universe.
- ○ Untapped creativity can cause blockages in our system.
- ○ Creativity requires that we stop chasing perfection and embrace self-acceptance.
- ○ Living a more creative life brings more joy into our lives.

CHAPTER TWELVE

Honouring Your Path

"*We are hungry. We are hungry for approval, attention, affection. We are hungry for the freedom to embrace life and to really know and be ourselves*"

EDITH EGER

Stepping into my role as a yoga teacher was daunting at first. I had imposter syndrome, lacked confidence, and never felt like I knew enough to begin teaching others. I was worried about what other people would think of me. But when the opportunities come knocking, we sometimes have to take a leap of faith and just go for it. When I first started teaching, I tried to imitate all the wonderful teachers I had experienced. I wanted to be just like them. I remember at one point even changing my accent to sound like my lovely teacher Tara from London. In time, as my confidence grew with practice, I found my own voice and my unique style of teaching.

We may never feel fully ready to step into our power. Our desire to be perfect and to do everything right can stop us from ever starting. When I think back to my early classes, I can see mistakes I made – instructions I gave incorrectly but that were never harmful to others, just simple mistakes. We learn and grow and become better from our mistakes. When our intention comes from a place of wanting to serve and help others, we are supported by the universal energy of love and can touch the lives of others. As we align with our power and prepare to step into our purpose, opportunities will present themselves to show us that we are ready. This is the universe supporting us. It is divine timing. And there is a sense of ease with divine timing. We do not have to force anything or chase after opportunities. All we need to do is enjoy the preparation, practise sacred patience, and trust that the right opportunities will present themselves. Have faith that you will recognise them when they arrive.

Living authentically

It is good to live in pursuit of our purpose, using our gifts and being true to ourselves. It takes a lot of energy to try to be someone else – it is draining on our body, mind and spirit. When we resist or deny our authentic self, life can be difficult and painful. We can end up bitter and resentful that we didn't follow our deepest yearnings. Joy and contentment can feel out of reach when we live misaligned to our true nature. Our gifts are a soothing balm to the world – a medicine, if you like – and we owe it to ourselves and the world to dig deep and find the courage to express them.

Finding the courage to live purposefully is not easy, though. It may mean making hard decisions to live in a very different way than how we are living now. We might experience pushback from others. But we might also experience more freedom, joy and contentment in our life than ever before, along with a deep sense of peace that can come with answering the call of our soul. In the process, we may discover that we inspire others by simply being ourselves. But how do we find the courage to truly be ourselves?

We will not be everybody's cup of tea

We cannot please everyone, and we need to stop trying. We are not here to be liked by everyone and to seek their approval. We won't be everyone's cup of tea, and there are lots of different flavours of tea on the planet. Spending our lives worrying about what other people think of us takes us off course and makes us afraid to step into our power. Speaking our truth and living in a way that is purposeful can trigger and upset others, but if our intentions come from the heart, we cannot harm anyone. Expressing our divine gifts is not a hurtful act; on the contrary, it is a healing one.

Nevertheless, the process of change and transformation can be isolating. As you move closer to being the real version of you, it will challenge people's accepted ideas of who you are. As we know, the human nervous system is more comfortable with certainty. And like change, personal growth is uncertain. We do not know the outcome or where we are being led. This uncertainty is challenging for us but also for others. Our path might make them uncomfortable. They may feel threatened when they see us trying something new in midlife. We should try not to take this personally. The judgements and criticisms of others are products of their own sense of insecurity. It is about them, not us. It is good to let go of grudges, forgiving others and wishing them well. This is not always easy, and it can be lonely for sure. But we should continue to stay on course and tell *our* story, not other people's.

Comparing leads to self-doubt

Sometimes we are too busy looking at what everyone else is doing to complete the great work that we came here to do. Just as it is none of our business what others think of us, it is also not our business what other people are doing. Getting too concerned or wrapped up in the lives of others is another distraction that consumes too much energy that could be spent more wisely doing other things.

Comparison fuels self-doubt. It makes us feel like we are in competition with others. This brings us back into a scarcity mindset. To break this cycle, it is best that we focus on our personal journey and stay out of things that are not our business. One practical way to do this is to explore our use of social media. We have a choice in whom or what we follow or consume online. We can feel uplifted and inspired by what people are sharing and we can learn about new things, but if we find ourselves comparing and it diminishes our self-worth, then we can choose to stop watching. When we engage in social media, we need to make sure it is adding value to our journey and not inhibiting our inner work. We can then use the tools of technology wisely to keep us focused on our own path.

CASE STUDY: Jennifer was a 43-year-old stay-at-home mum with three children. Her youngest son, Ryan, has autism. Much of her time was consumed advocating for Ryan and taking him to after-school appointments for speech and language therapy and occupational therapy. Years ago, she trained as a masseuse, and she used massage therapeutically with Ryan as a tool to help him to regulate his emotions and to sleep better. Jennifer never felt confident enough to practise massage outside the home, describing herself as having low self-esteem and perpetually worrying about how others perceived her. She told me that she spent a lot of time scrolling on social media, but that afterwards she felt very envious of other people's lives. Physically, Jennifer was very uptight. A big focus of our work together was to help her feel looser and lighter in her body, using joint-freeing movements, dance and intuitive movement to let go of tightness and feel more freedom in her body. We also worked on her self-confidence. I suggested she take a break from social media and use the wasted screen time to focus on herself rather than on what other people are doing. She decided to keep a journal during this period and noted that she was spending more time dancing in her kitchen. She felt lighter in her body and mind. As she let go of blocks, new opportunities arose in her life. A group of families with children with autism invited her to work with them in providing therapeutic massage for their children. Although initially nervous, Jennifer felt ready for the challenge to use her skills to serve others. She found meaning and purpose in this work and now helps to train other parents to use massage with their children.

Mind our own business

When we have discovered tools that help us, we can be eager to share this knowledge with people we care about. Even if our intentions are for their greater good, our unsolicited advice might be unwelcome, and it could be interpreted by others as our pushing our beliefs onto them. It is not our role to tell anyone else what to do. Everyone is on their own journey. It is not up to us to deprive them of the lessons that their lived experiences are here to teach them. Although it is hard to stand by and watch our loved ones suffer, we can let them know that we are here to support them if they need us. Naturally, when there is a genuine curiosity and they are actively seeking our help, we should generously share what we have learned with others. But we should not allow the path of another to distract or divert us from our own.

Do you trust that your gifts matter?

Often, the biggest barrier in our way is our own self-doubt. We can overcome all the other obstacles in our path once we trust that we are here to contribute something sacred. We might need a big shift in our old ideologies to truly believe that we have something valuable to offer the world and that our wisdom can make a difference to others. As we move into this next phase of our lives, we are called to shed our old perceptions of ourselves. This is a chance for rebirth, to step into our power. However, if we hold on to old judgements, then we limit ourselves. To build our confidence, we must let go of all the ideas that no longer serve us. Even after we have awoken to our purpose and our gifts, if we hold on to old ideas of ourselves and patterns of negative self-worth, they will stop us expressing our light.

PRACTICE: Burning ritual

Agni in yoga is described as the fire of transformation. We can use the heat of fire to burn off things that no longer serve us. This is a powerful ritual for releasing and letting go in order to welcome in change. We can burn away the impressions that no longer serve us, creating great change and transformation in our lives. For this practice, we will create a ceremony with fire to transmute whatever is getting in the way of your living purposefully.

Find a time and place where it is safe for you to create a little fire — even just the flame of a candle will do — with somewhere fireproof to burn some paper. You can create an atmosphere with soft music and scents. When you are ready, use a pen and paper and begin to journal what old beliefs are holding you back from living purposefully. This might include negative thoughts or biases that you hold about yourself or others, deeply buried fears, or even guilt that you don't deserve to fulfil your sacred potential. Put down everything you can think of that might be blocking you. After you are finished, fold the paper or tear it into small pieces. Find a safe way to burn these pieces of paper, either in your home fire or outside. As you watch the paper turn to flames, inhale a deep breath, and on the exhale, feel yourself releasing these blocks from your mind, body and spirit. Take a few breaths like this until you feel yourself getting lighter, no longer weighed down by these old patterns.

Trust that we have everything inside of us

When we trust that there is growth and lessons in all changes and new experiences, then we can surrender and let go. Deeply painful experiences often offer the biggest opportunities for us to gain perspective, clarity and wisdom. Life is a journey of navigating these experiences, some of which are more painful than others.

Buddhists teach that pain and suffering are unavoidable in life, but that it is how we react to our pain that determines whether we cause ourselves more suffering. The Buddha used a parable of two arrows. He said that we have two arrows coming our way in life. We can't always control the first arrow. This is the unavoidable pain and suffering. But the second arrow represents our reaction to the first.[1] This is the arrow that we can control.

It is important to honour the difficulties that we face in our lives, accepting the waves of feelings and emotions that arise from our challenging experiences, but also being open to the possibility that in time great learning can come from great pain. Fyodor Dostoevsky wrote: 'Pain and suffering are always inevitable for a large intelligence and a deep heart.'[2] When we see life as a school with lessons to teach us, we can recognise our challenges as opportunities for learning. This does not belittle the pain that we endure. The pain is unavoidable, but we can lessen the impact of our second arrow when we ask what this suffering is here to teach us. Reframing our pain can allow us to experience post-traumatic growth. Do we shy away from truly living and loving out of fear that one day we might experience loss? Or can we embrace all the opportunities and experiences in our life with courage, knowing that we have an inner warrior within each of us to help us through difficult times?

Be thankful to all our teachers

Some of the greatest wisdom in our lives comes from the challenging relationships we experience over our life course. Many Eastern traditions that believe in reincarnation also propose that we enter into soul contracts with other souls before we are born, agreeing to incarnate in order to help these souls learn lessons in this lifetime. Whatever your belief on incarnation, perhaps you can think of a time in your life when a teacher showed up to fuel your growth.

It is my experience that there is divine timing as to when these teachers show up. As the Buddhist and Taoist saying goes, 'when the student is ready, the teacher appears'. When we are ready, the teacher shows up in our life. It may be in the form of a romantic partner, friend or mentor. These relationships can challenge us to evolve and grow. Sometimes the relationships are short-lived, but if we receive the lesson, the wisdom remains for a lifetime. This can help us to accept the transient nature of some of our relationships. Leaning into the lessons, we find strength to trust that there is a greater plan for us and that everything is leading us to where we need to be. Then we can be thankful for all the teachers we have met along the way.

PRACTICE: Dropping into the well of wisdom within

Use this meditation any time you need to remind yourself that you have an abundance of courage and wisdom within you. Sit in a comfortable position. Allow your spine to elongate. When you are ready, begin to allow the breath to flow in through your nose and out through pursed lips as if blowing into a straw. Close your eyes if it feels OK to do so. Allow the awareness to come to the base of your spine. Visualise a deep well of wisdom at the base of your spine, also known as the root chakra. Imagine this well connected to the top of your head by a tube running the length of your spine, passing through all seven chakras. If you like, you can imagine the well of wisdom as being like a golden pond. Every inhale is a chance to gather wisdom in the form of a golden stream of light and allow it to move up the spine, illuminating your whole being. With every exhale through the mouth, feel the golden light leave the body and travel further and further into the distance, offering your wisdom into the world. Every inhale is a chance to gather more wisdom from the well and feel the light of wisdom moving up the spine. Every exhale is a chance to release this wisdom into the world and let go.

Allow this wisdom from your own well to nourish and guide you. Feel its divine energy filling up every space in your being. This is the same divine energy and intelligence that permeates nature. This natural intelligence is within you and all around you. Welcome this energy. Receive its wisdom, stay open, fill your cup — your whole being — with this wisdom, and release it through your exhale to serve the greater good. This is sacred wisdom that is available in abundance. It can nourish you and those around you. Spread your wisdom for the greater good. Radiate this light. Let us see the light in all beings. When you feel ready, allow your breath to return to its normal flow. Bring your hands together at your heart and bow to the light inside you.

Cultivating courage

Embracing our own light in midlife and beginning to allow others to see our potential takes courage and vulnerability. There will be times where we feel like we need to hide our light and step back into the shadows where our light is invisible. In these moments, we are overcome with fear. However, whatever we fear has no real power over us when we have true acceptance and love for ourselves. Usually, our fears are based on a perception of future events rather than a lived, present experience.

True courage is when we are aware of our fears, recognising and acknowledging them but not allowing them to stop us moving forward. When we are kind, loving and compassionate towards ourselves, we can handle fear of rejection, of unkindness or of being ridiculed, because we don't need outside acceptance or validation of our worth when we have an ever-present well of support internally. Our energy can be used in a much more enriching way when we connect to love rather than fear. Courage is within us all. To access it, however, we must first know that it is there. We might not always be aware of it or feel courageous, but within each of us there is a warrior. We can draw on this warrior strength, resilience and intuition to help us find the courage to live in a way that feels authentic for us. There is no need to look for courage outside of ourselves. When we come to trust the warrior within, we know the depth of strength that is available. Sometimes, we just have to believe it.

We cannot be afraid to make mistakes

We are each carrying wounds that manifest in different ways. When we are in pain, some of us externalise it, gossiping, critiquing others or lashing out and trolling online. This might offer us a temporary reprieve from our own pain, but it doesn't ultimately help our healing, and can actually compound our pain with the feelings of guilt that arise after our negative actions or comments. Many of us internalise the pain, trying to disguise it or bury it. Keeping our pain inside solidifies it, causing anger and bitterness. Our unresolved pain blocks us from connecting with who we truly are.

We are witnessing the manifestations of our collective pain in the divisiveness present in the world. With a very dichotomous view of right and wrong, many have become very unforgiving. We can be quick to criticise, punish and 'cancel' others for mistakes or errors in judgement. The growth of cancel culture spreads fear among many, which risks creating a threatening environment for self-expression. Self-expression must, of course, be informed and sometimes limited by the moral and legal responsibility to protect the human rights of others. There needs to be a balance between freedom of expression and the duty to protect others from harm, but if we always fear unintentionally offending others by saying the wrong thing, it sometimes becomes safer to say nothing.

We are all imperfect and have flaws – we will all make mistakes at some point in our life. It takes courage to admit mistakes, but mistakes are important opportunities for dialogue, learning, growth and forgiveness. This is not about advocating or remaining silent in the face of hateful speech, but rather about understanding that awareness, conversation, education and empathy are the keys to change. Shutting down voices is not always progress. It may at times serve to inflame and escalate hate and violence. When we push people to the margins, it is polarising and divisive – leading to the formation of extreme groups. This does nothing to unify the human race. Can we instead become compassionate listeners and allow space to hear opinions that are different from ours without feeling threatened? This would allow us to have meaningful discussions and conversations and create opportunities for each of us to learn and grow, while of course calling out and speaking up against anything that promotes hate and discrimination.

We are not here to fit in; we are here to change the old story

It is common, just before great transformation, to experience a whole range of emotions and inner turmoil. Often, this is described as the dark night of the soul. It can be as though we have been running a marathon only to hit the wall. As our awareness expands, our perception shifts and we uncover our truth. This can lead to changes in our life, our relationships and our friendships. Just like a death before rebirth, shedding our old ways of thinking and being in the world is necessary before we can emerge anew. But as we let go of what no longer serves us, we may experience resistance. Afraid of change and the uncertainty of what is ahead, we may decide to stick with the old, because at least it is familiar.

Although the process of metamorphosis can be hugely uncomfortable, things often need to get worse before they can get better. Like for a mother labouring her baby, the transition can be the most intense and painful stage. This is the moment when we are just on the cusp of birthing our greatness. But it is also a critical juncture, because it is the time when we most feel like quitting. Despite all our hard work and sacrifice, we can self-sabotage, feeling that we don't deserve to realise our potential. Paulo Coelho stated in the author's note to his fable *The Alchemist*: 'If you believe yourself worthy of the thing you fought so hard to get, then you become an instrument of God, you help the Soul of the World, and you understand why you are here.'[3] Knowing that we are here to have an impact on the world – not to fit in and play safe – can help us to find the final push to surrender to the process.

Find your support team

Ideally, mothers are never left alone to birth their babies. A whole team is involved, perhaps with a birth partner or doula, a midwife and doctors. We too need the support of a team to hold space for us during this transformational work of our midlife. Contrary to what we may have been conditioned to think, we don't have to do everything on our own. There are like-minded souls who understand the path we are walking. We need a hand to hold on this journey, providing us with some reassurance that it is safe to fully be ourselves.

The shared history that we have with family and old friends may not be enough to sustain us during this period of transition, however. They may mean well and want to offer solutions and advice when what we really need is to be heard. Furthermore, some may be triggered by our journey and unable to hold a safe space for us. Therefore, it is important to be open to new possibilities of support. We might need the professional support of therapists, doctors, healers and coaches.

We need to be patient – it may take time to find our team. We also need to be open to new people coming into our lives in the form of new acquaintances, new friends, new colleagues and new mentors who may be divinely appointed to support us at this stage of our journey. It is good to be receptive so that they can find us and we can recognise them as part of our team when they show up.

This genuine support may come in unlikely places. I came across the work of Niamh Gallagher, an intuitive energy healer, on Instagram during lockdown.[4] Her online sessions felt like soul therapy, and offered reassurance that I was not losing my mind during my own inner upheaval. My work with Niamh over the last few years gave me the clarity, insight and confidence to continue on my own path when fear and self-doubt crept into my mind. In the midst of great change and uncertainty, energy-healing modalities like reiki can help to clear resistance and leave us feeling earthed and grounded.[5] If you are feeling lonely on this path, trust that your community is coming, and seek out therapeutic support to anchor you while you feel at sea.

Ask for what you need

Don't be afraid to ask for what you need from those who love you. We cannot expect them to read our mind, yet we sometimes get resentful when they don't do what we need even though we have failed to ask or to express our needs. We must involve and include them in our journey in midlife, allowing them to support us by expressly asking for what we need. In my relationship, I have had to ask for more equal division of the childcare and domestic responsibilities so that I could have time to write this book. My partner was willing and able to cooperate. However, it took a little further work on my part to accept the support without imposing my way of doing things and being critical of the support.

Deepen our self-care practices

During the transition, as we shed layers of conditioning, we can feel exposed. It is unsettling, and we can feel like an outsider without a sense of belonging. In these moments of darkness, our fears will make us want to retreat back into the box of conformity. To stay on course, we need to empower ourselves to find ways to ground and replenish our reserves. Our self-care practices become our essential toolkit now.

It is important that we create uninterrupted time for our self-care and make this non-negotiable. I know a psychotherapist who schedules a session each day in her diary for herself to read, walk and fill her cup so she has something to give her clients. Retreats are great, but not practical or accessible for everyone. Little and often is more important. It doesn't require a huge chunk of time to incorporate a little self-care into your day. Be practical and realistic with what you do, and choose your self-care wisely to suit what you need. What works for one person might not work for another. See what you are called to try, and discover what is helpful for you at this time in your life.

We can, and I believe should, use different practices at different times in our monthly cycle, during different seasons and at different stages of our life. It is worth mentioning that it is totally normal that at challenging moments we may resist doing what we know is good for us. This is when we will really need to encourage ourselves to dig deep and use our self-care rituals. For example, the days that we don't want to move, walk or meditate may be the days we need those activities the most. What we resist persists, so it is good to have the awareness to know when we feel stuck and stagnant: this is when we need to change our energy and shift gears. You can return time and again to any of the practices in this book that felt useful to you.

Some examples of self-care are:

- Using physical movement to come back into your body
- Dynamic, gentle or restorative movement, depending on what you need
- Dancing to your favourite music to quickly shift your energy
- Taking a simple walk in nature – this can tick all the boxes for the body, mind and spirit, and the fresh air will oxygenate the body
- Resting if you are tired – sleeping, napping or using yoga nidra to replenish your energy
- Meeting a trusted friend for a catch-up
- Taking a relaxing bath with salts to ground and feel calm
- Using deep belly breaths to reassure your nervous system to find calm and safety
- Journaling to help release thoughts and fears onto the page
- Having a mindful moment to prepare and enjoy a hot drink
- Meditating on the breath to quieten the mind and find more clarity
- Seeking wisdom from spiritual books or podcasts that also inspire you

○ Getting creative and playful and doing things that
are fun to help you lighten up

We can trust in a higher power

No one can walk this path for us: we each have our own
unique journey. However, this does not mean that we
are alone. We can connect to a higher natural intelligence greater than us to guide and support us on our
voyage. Source energy is always available to us, if we
allow it, to recharge and refuel our tank when we feel
empty. When we trust that this energy is working for
our greater good, we can shift from fear to love, and
everything falls into place more easily. We can trust that
all is well and that all is as it should be in this present
moment.

How we develop this trust and faith will be unique
to each of us. I can only share with you how this has
evolved in my life. I have always had a deep sense of my
own destiny – an inner knowing – but I was so disconnected from myself that I did not trust myself to make
the decisions that served me best. As I have mentioned
in previous chapters, it felt easier for me to hand my
power over to others. However, about 15 years ago, the
day after my first date with my now husband, I experienced a deep, mystical experience that would take me
on a spiritual quest. I was shown a vision, like a home
movie projecting onto my bedroom wall. It showed
events that were to transpire in my life – my marriage,
my husband's career, and a boy aged about seven. I
also saw some images of relatives who had passed over

and others that would pass soon, with a comforting sense that they were all together. It felt like time stood still, even though it only lasted a couple of minutes. It seemed to me that there was a map to the order of my life that was prewritten and a destiny that was mine if I chose to follow it. This felt like evidence to me that a higher power was at work in the universe.

This mystical vision has helped me many times since to trust that everything is happening for my greater good. When I was pregnant with my first child, I was convinced that this was the boy I was shown in the vision. And when we found out during the pregnancy that the baby had a congenital heart defect and would need open heart surgery, I held firm that he would be okay because I had been shown him in the vision as an older boy. Woody had his operation at Great Ormond Street in London when he was only five months old. It was a worrying six hours of waiting, but I kept reminding myself of that image of him as an older boy, and it was so reassuring. I told my husband, 'Woody will be okay. He gets to be a bigger boy. I have seen it.' Since that experience, at times I have willed for more visions and mystical experiences, but it is my feeling that this desire blocks me from being receptive. It is in the non-effort that we are open to the grace of this divine power. I believe that these messages come in different mediums for different people. Author Susan Jeffers, in her book *Embracing Uncertainty*, writes about seeing a powerful healing light after her divorce that she felt was a higher power.[6]

CASE STUDY: Lara is a real-life local superhero.
She is a healthcare worker in one of the busiest
hospitals in Ireland. She uses her intuition to
make quick decisions that can save lives. She
deals with death every day and relies on her
connection to a higher power to support her
in her work. She is very humble about her
courage and bravery and only told me this
story after I brought up something similar
that was in the news. One night, as Lara was
coming home from her shift, a police alert
came on the radio to be on the lookout for
a car that had potentially been involved in a
crime. As the radio presenter called out the
details of the car model and registration, Lara
was stopped at a red light. She instantly looked
at the car in front of her and saw it was the
actual car they had just described. Without
hesitation, she rang the police and began to
follow the suspect. When I asked her if she
was afraid, she told me that she felt a divine
presence had come over her and she had
felt completely protected. Lara's bravery led
the police to the suspect, who had brutally
murdered a young woman. At the Coroner's
Court, Lara met with the victim's family, who
thanked her for her courage and acknowledged
that without her they would not have had any
answers about what happened to their beloved

daughter. I really believe that people like Lara
are earth angels and that they are here to
remind us that we can trust in a higher power.

Our greatest beauty is in showing up

As we clear out our old ways and overcome our self-
doubt, we find room to invite in more self-acceptance.
Accepting ourselves in our entirety – shadow and light
– is the path to self-confidence and allows us find new
ways of being in the world. We become secure in the
knowledge that it is OK not to know everything. We are
not a finished project. Right up until our last breath, we
have the potential to grow and learn. There is a great
mystery to life, and we will never know everything.

If we can accept this, we can stop hiding behind
everything we don't know, step into our role and start
sharing what we do know. If the flowers were afraid
to bloom, choosing to stay tightly closed, they would
deprive the world of their natural beauty. The same is
true for us. Our authentic self is our beauty. When we
allow ourselves to have the courage to fully bloom and
become who we are meant to be, we offer our beauty
to the world. Courage is an act of love. Retreating is
an act of fear. Courage leads us to growth and evolution. Retreating brings us towards self-protection, shutdown and decay. Choosing love is a display of courage.
Choosing the energy of love over fear and allowing our
authentic self to show up in the world is our gift to

the planet and our way of giving back to the universe. Showing up as our authentic self is the most courageous thing we can do.

PRACTICE: The Braveheart mudra

In the practice of yoga, *mudras* are hand gestures to invoke divine qualities. This mudra was taught to me by a great wisdom teacher, Michael McCann, from Belfast.[7] It invites us to have a courageous heart that is open and loving. Use this mudra whenever you want to connect to your brave heart and invite more courage into your life to help you overcome your fears.

Sit comfortably on a chair or a cushion. Bring your hands to your heart centre. Cross the right wrist in front of the left wrist. Allow the backs of the hands to touch. Now interlace the two little fingers together, then the two middle fingers together, and finally the index fingers together. Leave the ring fingers free. Then bring the tip of the right ring finger and right thumb to touch and bring the tip of the left ring finger and the left thumb to touch. Take a few breaths into your heart. Feel the space around your heart centre begin to expand and open. Welcome in the qualities of courage, strength and power into your heart. You might feel these qualities as a light or colour radiating from your heart.

Allow this light of courage to expand from your heart into your whole being. Remember that this sacred light is always inside you and was placed there to give you courage to express your unique gifts. The light is divine, and you can connect with it whenever you doubt that you have anything to offer this world. After the practice, take a moment to notice any whispers of guidance that you feel as you invoke the mudra. You may want to write down anything that you feel called to remember.

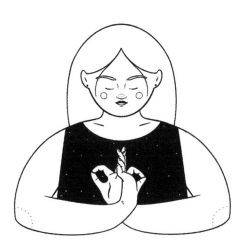

Pearls of wisdom

- ○ We should all live in pursuit of our purpose, using our gifts and being true to ourselves.
- ○ We owe it to the world to find the courage to express our gifts.

○ Stop comparing and worrying about what other people will think.

○ Stay focused on your own path.

○ Trust that your gifts matter and that everything you need is inside you.

○ Every experience is a chance to learn and grow.

○ We are here to have an impact on the world, not to fit in and play safe.

○ Deepen your self-care practices to cultivate strength and courage.

○ Showing up as our authentic selves is the most courageous thing we can do.

Epilogue

As you continue on your courageous journey towards, through and beyond midlife, my wish for you is that you can trust in the universe to know that you are fully supported to allow your gifts and wisdom to be shared generously with others. As you step into your wise power to live with more authenticity, meaning and purpose, you can inspire others to become the fullest expression of all they can be. Please come back to the practices in this book whenever you need self-nurturing and reminding of the wise woman that you are. As you awaken to the truest version of yourself, trust that we are all here on the earth in this moment to guide, teach and help one another to reach our wisest potential.

NOTES

CHAPTER ONE

1. Hubbard, J., Harbaugh, W. T., Srivastava, S., Degras, D., and Mayr, U. (2016). A general benevolence dimension that links neural, psychological, economic, and life-span data on altruistic tendencies. *Journal of Experimental Psychology: General, 145*(10), 1351–1135.

2. Maslow, A. H. (1993). *The Farther Reaches of Human Nature.* Penguin.

3. His Holiness the Dalai Lama reportedly made this statement at the Vancouver Peace Summit in September 2009.

4. Dorothy is the main protagonist in the *The Wizard of Oz,* a 1939 American musical fantasy film produced by MGM. Santiago is the main character in Coelho, P. (2006). *The Alchemist.* Harper Collins.

5. Yeats. W. B. (2001). *The Green Helmet and Other Poems.* Blackmask Online.

6. TEDx Talks. Crisis as a turning point: The gift of liminal time, Jean Shinoda Bolen, 23 April 2021, https://www.youtube.com/watch?v=9u3JZPCW9Dw.

7. Ibid.

8. Shinoda Bolen, J. (1986). *Goddesses in Everywoman*. Harper-Collins.

9. Ibid.

10. I have based these seven archetypes on the work of Jean Shinoda Bolen and the work of Niamh Gallagher, an Irish intuitive and energy healer. Niamh works with feminine leadership archetypes and has created a quiz to discover your feminine leadership archetype. Take the quiz here https://niamhgallagher .com/feminine-archetypes-quiz/.

11. Rumi, J. (1995). *The Essential Rumi*. HarperCollins.

CHAPTER TWO

1. https://www.industryarc.com/Research/Anti-Aging-Market -Research-508406?gclid=CjoKCQjwwJuVBhCAARIsAOPw GARtCoevdSnqo3NCyDvP7YglTGLFzctMvP5Eq2F3kLPzojx ZoQ-aQhUaAvvTEALw_wcB.

2. Jung, C. (1954). *The Development of Personality*. Collected Works XVII. Routledge.

3. Brooks, A. (2022). *From Strength of Strength: Finding success, happiness and deep purpose in the second half of life*. Bloomsbury.

4. Maslow, A. H. (1993). *The Farther Reaches of Human Nature*. Penguin.

5. Freed, J. (2022). *A Map of Your Soul Using the Astrology of Fire, Earth, Air, and Water to Live Deeply and Fully*. Rodale Books

6. The dosha questionnaire has kindly been designed by Ratna Dey-Cordukes, a certified Ayurveda Practitioner based in London. To learn more about Ratna's work, see her website, https://forbalance.com.

7. NICE (2015). Guidelines on Menopause Management and Diagnosis, https://www.nice.org.uk/guidance/ng23.

8. European Menopause and Andropause Society, https://emas-online.org.

9. See https://patient.info/doctor/premature-ovarian-insufficiency-pro.

10. See https://rockmymenopause.com/get-informed/menopause/.

11. Chandler, J. (2021). Menopause around the world. See https://www.mindsethealth.com/matter/menopause-around-the-world.

12. Melby, M. K. (2005). Vasomotor symptom prevalence and language of menopause in Japan, *Menopause, 12*(3), 250–257.

CHAPTER THREE

1. See Thích Nhát Hanh's talk on taking care of yourself, https://www.youtube.com/watch?v=MlLvjFPtFXw.

2. Enders, G. (2014). *Gut: The inside story of our body's most underrated organ.* Ullstein Buchveralge GmbH.

3. Ibid.

4. Benson, H. and Klipper, M. Z. (1975). *The Relaxation Response.* Morrow.

5. Porges, S. W. (2011). *The Polyvagal Theory: Neurophysiological foundations of emotions, attachment, communication, and self-regulation.* W. W. Norton & Co.

6. Van der Kolk, B. (2014). *The Body Keeps the Score: Brain, mind, and body in the healing of trauma.* Viking.

7. Burke Harris, N. (2020). *Toxic Childhood Stress: The legacy of early trauma and how to heal.* Pan Macmillan.

8. Lipton, B. H. (2016). *The Biology of Belief: Unleashing the power of consciousness, matter & miracles,* 10th anniversary edition. Hay House, Inc.

CHAPTER FOUR

1. Brizendine, L. (2022). *The Upgrade: How the female brain gets stronger and better in midlife and beyond.* Hay House Inc.
2. Ibid.

CHAPTER FIVE

1. Deloitte (2022). Women@Work 2022: A global outlook, https://www2.deloitte.com/content/dam/Deloitte/global/Documents/deloitte-women-at-work-2022-a-global-outlook.pdf.
2. Sri Swami Satchidananda (1988). *The Living Gita: The Complete Bhagavad Gita – A commentary for modern readers.* Integral Yoga Publications.
3. Fukuoka, M. (1978). 'The One-Straw Revolution', in *The New York Review of Books.*
4. David, M. (1991). *Nourishing Wisdom: A mind–body approach to nutrition and wellbeing.* Harmony.
5. Watch Oprah Winfrey talk about the disease to please here: https://www.youtube.com/watch?v=fde6rbPJbxA.

CHAPTER SIX

1. Emmons, R. A. (2013) *Gratitude Works: A 21-day program for creating emotional prosperity.* Jossey-Bass.
2. O'Donohue, J. (1997) *Anam Cara: Spiritual wisdom from the Celtic world,* p. 147. Bantam Press.
3. Schwartz, R. C. (2021). *No Bad Parts. Healing trauma and restoring wholeness with the Internal Family Systems Model.* Sounds True.
4. Ibid.

CHAPTER SEVEN

1. O'Donohue, J. (1997). *Anam Cara: Spiritual wisdom from the Celtic world.* Bantam Press.
2. Cameron, J (1992). *The Artist's Way: A spiritual path to higher creativity.* Souvenir Press.
3. Winfrey, O. and Parry, B. (2021) *What Happened to You? Conversations on trauma, resilience, and healing.* MacMillan.
4. Bowlby, J. (1968). *Attachment and Loss, Vol. 1: Attachment.* Basic Books.
5. Maté, G. (2018). *In the realm of hungry ghosts: Close encounters with addictions.* Vermillion.
6. Lee, H. (1988). *To Kill a Mockingbird.* Grand Central Publishing.

CHAPTER EIGHT

1. Frates, B. (2021). *Paving the Path to Wellness Workbook.* Healthy Learning.
2. Fredrickson, B. (2014). *Love 2.0: Creating happiness and health in moments of connection.* Plume Penguin House.
3. Shapiro, S. (2020). *Good Morning, I Love You: Mindfulness and self-compassion practices to rewire your brain for calm, clarity, and joy.* Sounds True Inc.
4. Watch the clip of the interview here: https://www.youtube.com/watch?v=Mh4f9AYRCZY.
5. Luft J. and Ingham H. (1955). *The Johari Window: A graphic model for interpersonal relations.* University of California Western Training Lab.
6. Zukav, G. (1991). *The Seat of the Soul: An inspiring vision of humanity's spiritual destiny.* Rider.
7. Richardson, D. and McGeever, J. (2018). *Tantric Sex for the Menopause: Practices for spiritual and sexual renewal.* Destiny Books.

8. Shapiro, S. (2020). *Good Morning, I Love You: Mindfulness and self-compassion practices to rewire your brain for calm, clarity, and joy.* Sounds True Inc.

9. See http://www.usmagazine.com/celebrity-news/news/jane-fonda-at-74-i-have-never-had-such-a-fulfilling-sex-life-2012107#ixzz3XDbEHZiO).

10. Fredrickson, B. (2014). *Love 2.0: Creating happiness and health in moments of connection.* Plume Penguin House.

CHAPTER NINE

1. Miyazaki, Y. (2018). *Shinrin-yoku: The Japanese way of forest bathing for health and relaxation.* Hachette.

2. Ibid.

3. Porges, S. (2011). *The Polyvagal Theory: Neurophysiological foundations of emotions, attachment, communication, and self-regulation.* W. W. Norton & Co.

4. Liz Reilly is a Reiki Master and yoga teacher based in Co. Wexford, Ireland. To find out more about Liz's work see https://bhaktihealing.ie.

CHAPTER TEN

1. Buettner, D. (2008). *The Blue Zones: Lessons for living longer from the people who have lived the longest.* National Geographic Books.

2. For more on the VIA Institute, see https://www.viacharacter.org/surveys.

3. Coelho, P. (2006). *The Alchemist.* HarperCollins.

4. García, H. and Miralles, F. (2017). *Ikigai: The Japanese secret to a long and happy life.* Hutchinson.

CHAPTER ELEVEN

1. Cameron, J. (1992). *The Artist's Way: A spiritual path to higher creativity.* Souvenir Press.
2. Osho (2011). *Creativity: Unleashing the Forces Within.* MacMillian.
3. Buettner, D. (2008). *The Blue Zones: Lessons for living longer from the people who have lived the longest.* National Geographic Books.
4. World Economic Forum. *Top 10 Skills for 2025,* https://www.weforum.org/agenda/2020/10/top-10-work-skills-of-tomorrow-how-long-it-takes-to-learn-them/.
5. Suzuki, N. (2021). *Wabi-Sabi: The Wisdom in Imperfection.* Tuttle Shokai Inc.
6. Watch the clip of the interview here: https://www.youtube.com/watch?v=PHiuQLs7kgU
7. Donoghue, E. 'Emma Donoghue: "I have only from 8.30am to 3.30pm to work. It's a very healthy discipline."' *The Guardian,* 22 February 2018. https://www.theguardian.com/books/2017/jan/07/writing-day-emma-donoghue.

CHAPTER TWELVE

1. Thích Nhất Hạnh (1999). *The Heart of the Buddha's Teaching: Transforming suffering into peace, joy and liberation.* Riders.
2. Dostoevsky, F. (1866). *Crime and Punishment.* Penguin Classics.
3. Coelho, P. (2006). *The Alchemist.* HarperCollins.
4. Niamh Gallagher is an energy healer, intuitive guide and spiritual business mentor. Find out more about Niamh's work here: https://niamhgallagher.com.
5. Reiki is a Japanese form of energy healing founded by Mikao Usui.
6. Jeffers, S. (2003). *Embracing Uncertainty.* Hodder & Stoughton.

7. Michael McCann is a yoga and wisdom teacher in Belfast. He has been studying the ancient spiritual texts since the 1970s, and he is widely considered to be Ireland's preeminent yoga philosopher. You can find more about his work here: https://www.facebook.com/theyogawellni.

ACKNOWLEDGEMENTS

I would like to thank all of the people who helped bring this book to life.

Firstly, a massive thank you to Sarah Liddy, commissioning editor at Gill Books, for taking a gamble on me and believing in this book. My sincere thanks to Rachel Thompson and Gráinne Treanor for your skilful work in editing the text; and thank you to Tara O'Brien for your beautiful illustrations and to all the design team at Gill for bringing beauty to the pages.

Richie Sadlier, thank you for time and advice at the very early stages of this project. My deep thanks to my dear friend Ratna Dey Cordukes for the wisdom and insight you so generously gave to me and for allowing me to include some of your ayurvedic work in this book. Niamh Gallagher, I am forever grateful for your mentorship, intuitive guidance and for helping me to trust myself to birth this book. Dr Jackie Ang, thank you for your input on the early drafts of this book. Dr Natalie Summerhill, thank you for providing advice and support on the medical aspects of this book. To Amy Cowley, thank you for all the proofreading and support pulling this book together. I couldn't have done it without your assistance.

To all my wise teachers in Ireland – Liz Reilly, Ciara Cronin and Michael McCann – and my mentors at the wonderful Yoga Therapy Institute in the Netherlands – Monsterratt G, Caroline Kila and Marlene Jansen – thank you all for imparting your wisdom and teaching me how to hold space for other women. To Mary Francis Drake at Ubiquity University, I am so glad that the universe guided me towards your wise mentorship just as I was finishing this manuscript.

To all my wonderful clients: thank you so much for trusting me to support you in your practice. Thank you to all the women who allowed me to share their stories in this book. Thank you to all my friends, the wise women in my life past and present, for your meaningful connections. A special thank you to my dear friend Siobhan Byrne, for your kind words of encouragement on our dog walks together. Louise Shearer, thank you for boosting my confidence in my creativity and willing me on with this book.

To Mary Harris, my first wise woman, thank you for being my mother and my greatest cheerleader. To my dad, John, thank you for always being my guru and encouraging me to see different perspectives. To Ayshea and Lindsey, my sisters, thank you for your wise words when I need them most, even if I don't always seem like I am listening. Thank you to my children, Woody and Darcy, for your astounding patience and all the matcha lattes you got me while I was typing away. I love you both. Finally, thank you Dd for your love, encouragement and the reminders to keep smiling. *Maktub*.